ALL IN

Using Healthcare Collaboratives to Save Lives and Improve Care

Edited by:
Bruce W. Spurlock, M.D.
Patricia A. Teske, RN, MHA

With chapter contribution by:
Donald M. Berwick, M.D.

All In: Utilizing Healthcare Collaboratives to Save Lives and Improve Care Bruce Spurlock, M.D. and Patricia Teske, RN, MHA Eds.

Cynosure Health
1688 Orvietto Drive, Roseville, CA 95661

Books may be purchased by contacting the publisher and editors at:
Cover and Interior Design: Book Cover Cafe
Publisher: Ingram Spark
Printer: Ingram Spark

Editors: Bruce Spurlock, Patricia Teske
Creative Consultant: Arian Dasmalchi, ImageWorks Marketing & Communication

ISBN: 978-0-9967927-0-7
First Edition
Printed in USA

Contact: bspurlock@cynosurehealth.org; pteske@cynosurehealth.org
Website: www.cynosurehealth.org

10 9 8 7 6 5 4 3 2 1

CONTENTS

The Thing Speaks for Itself

By Patricia A. Teske, RN, MHA, Implementation
Officer, Cynosure Health

It was a very small community hospital—so small that I missed it and drove right by on my way to my job interview. I was hired to help develop a rehabilitation program, which was one of many last-gasp efforts to keep the failing hospital afloat. Within several months of my arrival, which was back in the day when The Joint Commission sent you a letter letting you know they were coming, the then director of quality decided to retire. I was sitting in a conference room with a dozen or so others when the CEO looked around the table. I was much younger then and didn't know to look down. So he looked at me and I looked back, and that's how I became the new director of quality.

Although I was flattered that the CEO thought I could do the job, my confidence rapidly plummeted when I realized that I knew very little about the position and my numerous new responsibilities. It was a small hospital and no one was there to show me the ropes. I reached out to any source I could find to help guide my journey, but few people were readily available. Those early days of struggling, and the help and mentoring I received from others, instilled in me the desire to support and mentor others as my career progressed.

About a month into my new role I was greeted in the parking lot by the CEO's administrative assistant. She said, "I'll park your car. You need to go inside." Knowing what I know now, I probably should have put my car into reverse and driven back home; but remember, I was much younger then.

Waiting for me was the lead physician from the county's department of health. She was there to investigate what was a precursor to an Emergency Medical Treatment and Active Labor Act (EMTALA) violation. A physician at my hospital had instructed a pregnant woman to drive to another local hospital before being examined. Although both the mother and baby had good outcomes, the potential for harm existed. The hospital received a lengthy report from the state for which an action plan was necessary. Due to my inexperience, I didn't know all of the regulations or how to comply with them, nor did I have a ready resource to guide me. This early experience left with me a strong desire to share my own experiences and learn from others. After several visits and too many hours of work to count, the matter was successfully resolved. There's nothing like on-the-job training, but I needed more.

I purchased cassette tapes that contained all the regulations so I could play them in my car. Not surprisingly, my children never wanted to drive anywhere with me. I was forlorn when a course I'd located for new quality professionals was cancelled due to lack of registration. I joined professional organizations and fortunately met others who were more experienced. Their mentoring and sheer perseverance enabled me to accomplish the job at hand.

Several years later, I left this small hospital and joined a larger one. From there I became the administrative director of quality over two merging hospitals. That position led me to become the vice president of quality and care management for what is now Dignity Health. From there I launched out independently and have had the great fortune of working on many quality and safety projects including BEACON, the Bay Area Patient Safety Collaborative.

Between 2005 and 2010, the Gordon and Betty Moore Foundation, a foundation dedicated to improving the environment, science and patient safety, funded the BEACON collaborative in the San Francisco Bay Area (SFBA) and the development of this book. The design and execution of BEACON was a partnership between the Hospital Council of Northern and Central California, the regional affiliate of the California Hospital Association;

and Cynosure Health, a non-profit quality improvement organization. BEACON's initial focus was on recruiting and supporting SFBA hospitals to participate in the Institute for Healthcare Improvement's national "100,000 Lives Campaign." In doing so, BEACON became one of the exemplar national "nodes" of this campaign and an early blueprint for other hospital collaborative efforts in the U.S.

Among the key design and implementation elements of BEACON were the following:

- A regional identity to inspire SFBA hospitals to work together towards regional improvement goals
- A focus on most significant harms in terms of mortality and morbidity
- A consensus prioritization among participants on which harms to address
- Aspirational (but realistic and evidence-based) goals with written commitment by the hospital CEO and/or hospital board
- These design elements were supported by:
    In-person meetings with significant peer-to-peer learning opportunities
    Deep dives into target improvement areas
    Discussions with national experts in the targeted clinical areas
    A focus on effective, efficient ways to implement the latest evidence at the bedside through on-the-ground hospital implementers sharing their tactics with their peers
    The provision of onsite technical assistance to participating organizations

Additionally, capacity for performance improvement was increased through quality improvement skill-building courses. Data collection of process and outcome measures, with personalized reporting to individual hospitals to highlight successes and areas of opportunity, was also used throughout the collaborative.

The resulting design elements and strong leadership of BEACON resulted in impressive outcomes, including active participation by 100 percent of SFBA adult acute care hospitals with greater than 83 percent of SFBA hospitals significantly improving care. They demonstrated this by achieving improvement targets in multiple clinical areas, including more than 1,000 lives saved.

Due to this impact, Anthem Blue Cross partnered with the National Health Foundation and California's Regional Hospital Associations in 2010 to independently fund the Patient Safety First initiative that incorporated many of elements of BEACON. Anthem Blue Cross and their regional hospital association partners even received the 2013 John M. Eisenberg Patient Safety & Quality Award, a national award by the National Quality Forum for their work on the Patient Safety First initiative.

There has been recent discussion in literature about how to determine the effectiveness of the learning collaborative, as will be discussed in several chapters of this book by Don Berwick and others. However, we believe it's self-evident that we can learn more from each other more rapidly than we can learn individually. We also believe that it's essential for learnings from large-scale learning collaboratives to be codified to be used in the future by other designers, implementers, funders and evaluators of collaborative efforts. To this end we've assembled an international group of advisors and contributors who have generously contributed to this book.

Throughout this book, we use the term "collaborative" to broadly define a group of organizations or individuals who are learning and working together towards a common aim. This multi-directional learning differentiates collaboratives from other types of activities in which learning is one-way. Other terms frequently used for this type of activity include "learning collaborative," "quality improvement collaborative" and "healthcare improvement collaborative." For simplicity's sake, we will adopt the term "collaborative" for all.

Also, this book is intended to describe a variety of approaches to designing, running and funding collaborative efforts. We don't believe there's just one way to learn together. Over time, collaboratives have been designed by numerous organizations to address various healthcare challenges. While the goal of improving healthcare is a common thread, the specific characteristics and structure of each collaborative vary, sometimes dramatically.

Characteristics that differentiate collaboratives include:

- Sponsorship type:
  - Condition-specific organizations focused on promoting and improving health related to a specific set of related health or disease conditions by serving as a resource of information, evidence-based best practices and guidelines. These organizations are often specialty organizations such as American Heart Association, American Stroke Association and California Maternal Quality Care Collaborative.
  - Medical specialty and professional organizations representing and supporting their members in areas of advocacy, and establishing professional standards and guidelines, education and resources, such as: American College of Obstetrics and Gynecology, Society of Hospital Medicine and American College of Cardiology
  - Improvement organizations whose mission is focused on improving patient safety, healthcare outcomes and population health, such as: The Institute for Healthcare Improvement, Regional Healthcare Improvement Organizations, Institute for Clinical Systems Improvement and Quality Improvement Organizations
  - Trade/sector organizations representing and supporting their members in areas of advocacy, policy, legislative and regulatory issues, such as American Hospital Association's Health Research and Educational Trust, State Hospital Associations and America's Health Insurance Plans

- Government or national, such as the Centers for Medicare & Medicaid Services and The Agency for Healthcare Research and Quality or state public health departments
- Other stakeholders such as Premier, Inc. a healthcare improvement alliance of 3,400 U.S. hospitals and 110,000 other providers, Press Ganey and Cardinal Health

- Association with registry/database, which can accelerate change through shared data by having advantages such as: 1) current participants already have the infrastructure and commitment to submit data, 2) pre-established dataset, 3) ability to analyze existing data to identify opportunities for improvement across the cohort, 4) ability to determine current organizational performance as a baseline as well as throughout the collaborative and 5) ability to provide comparative performance results. Examples include:
  - The Northern New England Cardiovascular Disease Study Group, a regional consortium founded in 1987, provided proof of concept that like organizations can work collaboratively to improve care.
  - Vermont Oxford Network, a nonprofit voluntary collaboration focused on neonatal care
  - American College of Surgeons National Surgical Quality Improvement Program, focused on preventable surgical complications, such as surgical site infections
  - National Cardiovascular Data Registry (NCDR), the American College of Cardiology's suite of cardiovascular data registries
  - Other emerging registries such as group purchasing organizations (e.g., Premier, VHA), regional and state databases (e.g., All Payer Claims Database, Wisconsin Healthcare Quality Collaborative) and many other professional, commercial and data-sharing organizations

- Funding sources: Includes internal funding by the sponsoring organization and external funding via contracts, grants or gifts. Participation fees may be used to offset some expenses.

- Single- vs. multiple-topic: Collaboratives sponsored by condition-specific organizations and registries most commonly identify a single clinical topic for improvement. The Institute for Healthcare Improvement's Breakthrough Series and Collaboratives also focus on a single topic. Other collaboratives provide a set of topics and allow participants to either select those topics of most importance to their organizations, or may require participants to work on all available topics.

- Time-limited vs. network/community: Collaboratives commonly seek to achieve improvement within a specified timeframe, usually defined by the sponsor and/or funding source. Others are not constrained by time and seek to create a community/network of collaboration such as the various Regional Health Improvement Collaboratives.

- Participating organizations: Hospitals/specific-care settings vs. multi-stakeholder participants. The profile of collaborative participants will be largely driven by the topic focus of the collaborative, overall purpose of the collaborative, the topic(s) to be addressed, as well as the sponsoring organization. Target participants are typically identified in the collaborative design phase.

- Learning delivery approach (in-person conferences/meetings, virtual, webinars, other): The learning approaches will vary from collaborative to collaborative and will be driven by factors such as funding and proximity.

- Campaign approach: Certain characteristics of a political campaign mirror what healthcare leaders seek to achieve, with campaign professionals working with firm targets (the number of votes needed to win) and a firm deadline (election day). Campaigning results in organizing actions around a specific issue, seeking to bring about change, and mobilizing individuals to influence others to affect desired change.

- Internally vs. externally sourced: Decisions regarding who will administer the collaborative and who will support the collaborative topic content development and delivery will be made during the planning and design phase. The decision to source internally or externally will likely be driven by the sponsoring organization's capacity and capability.

    Early on in the process we held advisory group calls and interviewed potential end users of this work. Throughout this book we've brought together a variety of contributors who represent diverse perspectives ranging from the original IHI breakthrough series to enduring communities of improvement. The variation in approach is on display throughout the book, yet common themes emerge:

- Basic building blocks are necessary for all collaborative improvement work. These are described throughout the book and include such items as selecting an appropriate intervention and target population, creating a concrete and bold aim, data collection, submission and reporting with actionable measures, flexible operational elements, peer-to-peer exchange, growing improvement capabilities, and building relationships around an identity bigger than yourself or your organization.
- The ability to adapt while running a collaborative is also a core success feature. Adapting an intervention for different environments, refocusing energy towards unanticipated challenges, adjusting measures if they become a barrier, and many other details need continual fine-tuning almost from the outset.
- Collaborative leaders need to address both the group as well as the individual dynamics. Are the leaders engaged? Are problems being shared among the participants?
- Bringing together multiple perspectives and using contemporary evaluation methods along with rigorous improvement science leads to continual innovation in designing and running collaboratives.

The book is meant to be a guide. It sets forth what's been learned, overcoming challenges, facing barriers and suggesting areas where additional knowledge is needed on a variety of topics encountered by those designing, running and funding collaborative efforts. It's not a research-driven book, although research is cited throughout the text. The numerous contributors share their broad and diverse experiences from different settings, on different topics so that the cumulative effect speaks for itself. While the experiences and opinions they share are their own and are not attributable to the editors nor the Gordon and Betty Moore Foundation, they enrich the book and support innovation and creativity in designing and running a collaborative. It's arranged in chapter segments so that it can be used in its entirety or in modular format.

It makes sense to learn from the experiences of the past. Our goal with this book is to help shape the future of learning collaboratives by experimenting and sharing with other collaborative leaders so that future collaboratives won't need to struggle when knowledge that could help you exists but isn't readily accessible. Additionally, the book is a call to action to help shape the future of learning collaboratives by experimenting and sharing with other collaborative leaders.

Going back to my initial story... although I was flattered that the hospital CEO thought I could be the director of quality, I was woefully unprepared for my role. Fortunately, I was able to reach out and learn from others enabling me to work in this field of patient safety and quality improvement for several decades. I can't imagine a more fulfilling way to spend my professional career.

This book's title, "All In: Using Healthcare Collaboratives to Save Lives and Improve Care," reflects the notion that we'll all improve faster if we work collaboratively. We believe that it speaks for itself that learning together is better than learning alone. Are you all in?

CHAPTER 1

Accelerating Change at Scale: Spreading Effective Practices

By Joe McCannon
System Spread vs. National Spread by Jason Byrd, J.D.

"I think when people look back at our time, they will be amazed at one thing more than any other. It is this — that we do know more about ourselves now than people did in the past, but that very little of this knowledge has been put into effect."

—Doris Lessing

Introduction

On a bitterly cold February day in 2010, I went to a distinguished Boston hospital to pick up my uncle. He had just had a serious surgery, and after almost a week of recovery and rehabilitation, he was judged ready to return home.

I collected his belongings and the discharge papers that were scattered on his bedside table. I had just finished a decade of work in patient safety, so I asked him if he was clear on the instructions, particularly regarding his new medications.

"Not really," he told me. A long-time Boston police officer and a one-time force of nature, he looked tired and shaken.

"OK," I said, "is there someone we can talk to about that?"

He shrugged. I found a nurse in the hallway and asked for her help.

"I already talked about that with him," she told me.

"I don't think he's clear on it," I explained, and she returned with me to the room.

"You understand your meds, hon?" she asked him.

"Well, mostly," he replied, smiling. "But could you repeat what you said to my nephew?"

She rattled off a list of five medications and when he should take them. As she spoke I tried to follow along in his discharge plan, reviewing two forms— one typed and one handwritten—that contained some of what she said and contradicted other parts of it. I pointed out the discrepancies.

"Don't worry about that," she said, gesturing at the papers. "Just do what I said and you'll be all set."

"I'm not sure I can remember what you said," I told her.

"But you can, right, hon?" she said to my uncle. He nodded and smiled, and she began to back out of the room.

"Wait, are his prior medications included here?" I asked.

"Yes, they should be," she said. She turned to my uncle, "All your old meds are included on the list, right?"

He nodded and smiled again.

I wasn't so sure.

He insisted that we leave, though, and against my better judgment, I assented.

On the drive home, I was anxious. I wasn't sure that we had a complete or correct medication list, and I wasn't sure where I was going to get the answers I required. Ultimately—after almost 24 hours of politely pestering assorted physicians, nurses and pharmacists—my mother and I got a satisfactory medication list.

While the experience bewildered and frustrated me, I share it mainly because of the realization I had two days later when I was reflecting on the incident. I had seen a superb example of medication reconciliation only a few months earlier, and it had occurred not in another part of the country, not in another part of the state, not in another local system but in the same hospital. It was astonishing.

Despite my interest in variation in cost and quality in the American healthcare system, despite years studying at the knee of Don Berwick and Jim Conway and a whole host of luminaries in the field of patient safety, I suddenly felt the impact of reality in a much more visceral and personal way. Variation in quality in American healthcare is not merely "interesting," "troubling" or "worthy of deep research;" it's fundamentally unjust. When we know how to do something that can save lives or reduce suffering, and we fail to reliably make it available to anyone who could benefit, we're all at risk of seeing our loved ones subjected to avoidable harm. We can do better.

Spreading Knowledge Faster

The fact is that for nearly every known threat to our health and well-being— for nearly any social problem—a solution exists. We know, for instance, how to reduce carbon dioxide emissions. We know how to end chronic homelessness. We know how to rapidly improve literacy and high school graduation rates. Innovative models that get better results exist in pockets across the nation and around the globe.

This is especially true in healthcare. The research community continuously produces breakthrough biomedical innovations capable of saving many lives, and practitioners of care are themselves continuously innovating in care delivery in an attempt to better serve their patients. Obamacare, which demands significant change on many dimensions— including new approaches to managing population health, improvement in the quality of care and reductions in the cost of care—has only intensified the rate of innovation.

But while there's no shortage of new ideas in healthcare, the slow rate at which evidence-based practices spread to everyone who could benefit from them is troubling. Balas and Boren famously suggested that it takes an average of 17 years to implement sound research at the front lines of care.[1] Important studies on variation in quality and cost of care by Wennberg, Fisher and others underscore the point.[2,3,4] Our critical enterprise, then, is not merely discovery but taking what's known as rapidly as possible to everyone who could benefit from it. Addressing this challenge—identifying vehicles for spreading knowledge—has been a project of growing importance in the field in the last quarter century and forms the basis for this book.

A major insight in this period has been that traditional forms of dissemination don't work in changing behavior at scale. Publishing, presenting and developing websites—while of some value in raising awareness of innovations—aren't sufficient to lead to broad adoption of new practice. Nor does classroom-style teaching, for all of its familiarity, effectively transmit knowledge; passive learning of this kind rarely leads to meaningful behavior change.[5] Instead, we've come to understand that *distributed, networked hands-on learning*—where every targeted adopter a) becomes an active agent of local change and adaptation to make the new idea thrive in their setting, and b) actively studies and learns from the challenges and solutions of their peer organizations ("all teach, all learn," in the parlance of Institute for Healthcare Improvement)—is a more effective approach.

To spread a new practice, we can't merely teach or exhort others; we must unleash them to operate at their highest levels of creativity and intensity. We need to deliberately build a corps of motivated change agents arrayed across the area we seek to serve—curious, data-driven, avid for improvement and willing to share their ideas and their challenges. The benefits of this kind of empowerment and collaboration are striking. Participants apply new ideas, refine and improve upon them, and a much larger community, of colleagues and patients and families, benefits in turn.

The specific vehicles we can use for creating distributed, networked hands-on learning are several—campaigns, collaboratives, extension agency, wave sequencing and grassroots organizing, to name a few. All, however, contain some key similarities: They bring together many individuals or organizations in a network; they take expert-vetted content and seek to spread it to the group, encouraging local adaptation; they create a structure wherein participants regularly test new practices (and receive feedback on their progress); and they seek to facilitate exchange of practical knowledge among participants.

Importantly—and despite significant debate on the topic—there's no single "best" approach. Each is appropriate for different contexts at different moments in time. As seminal thinkers in the field such as Everett Rogers have noted, a number of factors require consideration in the selection of the right method for spreading effective practice[6]:

- **Nature of the innovation:** Are we introducing an innovation or practice that's thoroughly tested and well-established? Or are we still refining it? Is the practice in question straightforward (e.g., easy to introduce, located in a single setting)? Or is it more complex? Will we have to persuade people of its value? Or will its value be readily apparent?

- **Size and nature of the audience we seek to reach:** How many people do we need to reach if we are to bring our intervention to everyone who could benefit from it? What's the disposition of the audience we seek to reach? What's the disposition of key executives and opinion leaders? How does the audience break down on the continuum from "highly innovative" to "highly reluctant?" How much experience do they have in adopting new practices? How are they arrayed geographically? Which types of facilities do they represent?

- **Available resources and infrastructure:** Is there independent funding to support construction of the network? Do we need to build it organically, with no new resources? What kind of staff support is available to run the network?

Will we be able to bring people together in person? Will there be access to tools and technologies to connect people to one another?

- **Time frame to drive change:** How much time is available to spread the practice in question? Is it fixed? Is it mutable?

There are resources that address these factors while offering guidance on which approaches to spreading change are appropriate and when they should be applied, though more thorough treatments of this topic would be welcome.[7]

Coming Together Effectively

Of all of the previously mentioned approaches to spreading improvement, the collaborative is the one that's come onto the scene most forcefully in recent years. Pioneered by the Institute for Healthcare Improvement in the mid-1990s, it's become increasingly common as a way for non-profits, foundations, health plans and governments to bring together the healthcare providers and organizations they seek to reach with new innovations. Fields outside of healthcare like education and human services now use it as well.

In its generic form, a collaborative is usually a collection of healthcare organizations of a similar type that come together over a fixed period to pursue a shared and measurable improvement aim—perhaps reducing the rates of unneeded cesarean sections or reliably managing diabetes, for example. During the course of the initiative, they come together—sometimes in person, sometimes by phone or webinar—to report to one another on progress, sharing their challenges and offering one another advice. The collaborative provides a structure and rhythm (e.g., weekly conference calls might require participants to test new ideas and report on their progress each week) and creates shared expectations for improvement. In between, email lists, websites and online workspaces allow participants to ask questions, make notes on what's working and celebrate breakthroughs, big and small. Common tools allow participants to collect their data and array it over time, using the rules of statistical process control to identify meaningful changes in performance.

Many of the best examples of healthcare improvement I've witnessed came in collaboratives. I recall watching a collection of hospitals and clinics in a rural South African district came together in an attempt to rapidly expand access to antiretroviral treatment for HIV/AIDS, making remarkable progress within a matter of months. I think of Rashad Massoud's wonderful work across several large oblasts in Russia to improve neonatal outcomes.[8] I remember the wonderful energy and outcomes of Bay Area Patient Safety Collaborative, previously discussed in the introduction, which later became BEACON, totally transforming expectations about what's possible in patient safety across the entire region. At their best, these efforts build vibrant, generous and fun communities that facilitate rapid learning, creating lasting relationships and reusable infrastructures that they use to address other systemic problems in healthcare. Following is a case study from the Carolinas HealthCare System.

Case Study: System Spread vs. National Spread

By Jason Byrd, J.D.

Successfully driving improvement relies upon understanding and using key tactics relevant to your target audience. Much like politics, all collaboratives must be seen as local. If local organizations and frontline teams don't engage and execute, even the best learning collaboratives, whether national or local, ultimately fail. Though the tactics used by national and local efforts differ, common themes exist.

Leadership credibility is key to both national and local improvement initiatives, but it manifests itself in different ways. In national initiatives, leadership credibility is often related to the perspective, voice and reputation of an organization or individual. Organizations, such as Institute for Healthcare Improvement (IHI) and American College of Cardiology (ACC), have at least in part achieved success based on their ability to garner attention for their efforts. The attention is a byproduct of the reputations they've worked diligently to enhance among clinicians, administrators and policymakers. When credible organizations speak, collaborative participants listen.

Local improvement initiatives rely upon credible leaders in a different way. Successful local leaders bring their reputations, knowledge, and appreciation of local challenges and circumstances. They can engage provider organizations by translating national collaborative themes to a local impact. For example, as part of the Partnership for Patients Hospital Engagement Network (HEN) initiative, Carolinas HealthCare System found success in describing to an individual hospital how its harm reduction efforts feed into broader, national improvements to patient safety. In general, hospital teams are proud and excited to have their work and results seen by others across the nation. It's essential to understand the complexities of local resources, patient populations and environmental contexts, and develop appropriate implementation strategies for improvement.

All successful learning collaboratives, and leaders in general, possess a healthy dose of self-awareness. They understand their role to provide solid evidence, consensus recommendations, value-added resources (e.g., change packages, templates, guidelines) and individual leaders capable of engaging the heart and the mind. Two key leaders who embody these dynamics are Don Berwick, former CEO of IHI during the 100,000 Lives Campaign, and Harlan Krumholz, cardiologist at Yale University and leader of ACC's Door-to-Balloon (D2B) campaign.

Local efforts engage respected champions to further spread improvement and recognize the need to approach and engage one individual at a time. In addition, strong local data access affords opportunities to focus improvement efforts and accomplish broader national objectives. For example, understanding that patients with a sepsis or pneumonia diagnosis comprise the most significant portion of your readmission population provides better improvement opportunities than simply tackling a goal related to readmissions.

Finally, all successful collaboratives effectively use "unfunded mandates" to drive improvement. National efforts communicate to and convince audiences of the importance of significant issues (e.g., harm reduction, door-to-balloon times). They are the catalyst for a broader "movement" and cultural change, capitalizing on the readiness of the organizations, even when most won't have additional resources to accomplish the work. Many of these efforts use competitive peer pressure to increase participation, particularly as national collaboratives grow and gain media attention.

But unfunded mandates in local efforts are a more complex challenge. At the individual organizational level, they navigate challenging discussions related to lack of resources. Influence and persuasion are key attributes to overcoming these obstacles. Further, successful local efforts are flexible in their understanding of local dynamics and adapting national recommendations that drive improvement.

While the balance of this book goes into the specifics of how to design and instrument a collaborative, it's important to note that how the collaborative is managed—its leadership behaviors, its operating norms and its day-to-day cadence—is every bit as predictive of success as thoughtful strategy and design. A great deal of funding is squandered when it's invested in well-designed efforts that look good on paper but fail to see results across participating institutions. Devolving into a series of meetings or didactic webinar sessions, these are collaboratives in name only.

By contrast, the exceptional collaboratives mentioned previously are set apart by a spirit that animates all good work to spread change, regardless of the specific spread method selected. It's relentless, agile, data-driven and completely results-focused, and it truly empowers all participants to be active engines of change themselves.

Specifically, the following are the operating values that infuse large-scale improvement initiatives that succeed in getting better results:

- **Quantifiable aims that all participants share:** "Reduce medication errors" isn't an aim. Neither is "improve patient experience." To create real tension for change among participants in a collaborative, it's critical to have an aim that's explicit and time-bound. Knowing exactly what we seek to accomplish—by a specific date—raises the stakes on performance and gives us a sense of whether we're making meaningful progress. Moreover, we should expect every participant to meet the aim in their own setting, to make their contribution to the success of the overall group, creating shared accountability and additional incentive for collaboration. (Importantly, tracking measures is not the same as setting aims. Aims tell us what we aspire to, and commit to do, and measures allow us to assess our progress against those objectives.)

- **Engaged leadership that focuses on removing barriers:** The role of leadership—in those organizations orchestrating the initiative and in provider organizations—is critical. If leadership cares about the aim, those at the front lines of care who are charged with actually improving practice can feel that attention deeply. In addition, it's important that leadership signals a strong interest in empowering those practitioners through active support and involvement, rather than expecting reports on progress and creating fear by repeatedly exhorting and demanding results. They must visit the places that are delivering the care, understand impediments to success and use their.[8] One promising collaborative to reduce multi-drug resistant tuberculosis in and around Lima, Peru, institutionalized this role through a team of local leaders who convened regularly to understand obstacles in securing needed resources, drugs and supplies and rapidly addressed these obstacles[9]. Helping leaders to understand their proper role is a major enterprise of the collaborative. Many collaboratives require endorsement and regular participation from executives, for instance, while others go to great lengths to educate leaders on the human and financial costs associated with continued underperformance, as well as the benefits and opportunities created by improvement.

- **Thoughtful use of data:** Good and timely data is an essential and positive element of collaborative improvement work when it's used properly. Arrayed over time, with proper annotation, it gives participants a clear sense of whether they're making sustainable progress and offers clues as to the sources of meaningful improvement (or underperformance). But when we use data for comparison and judgment, it can lead to fear and dispute. Some hide disappointing results while others challenge what the data says. No one asks questions, and therefore no one learns. It's much better to ask participants to focus on how they're improving against themselves, zeroing in on their own rate of progress instead of worrying about comparative outcomes.

- **Rhythmic testing and adjustment (spirit of improvisation and learning):** In a surprising number of collaboratives, subject experts teach participants who have no obligation to actually test new interventions and practices themselves. The hypothesis, it seems, is that the participants will immediately adopt the lessons learned from these authorities. Everything we know about change management and quality improvement suggests that this is wishful thinking. A strong collaborative will not simply invite its participants to listen and passively absorb new information; rather it will insist that they apply new ideas and practices—testing them at a rapid rate—to adapt them locally and improve faster. They must become innovators and improvisers if they are to succeed in their own setting, where they will surely encounter local resistance and context-specific challenges. In this respect, traditional, summative evaluations that ask participants to adhere strictly to guidelines to avoid contamination of the experiment, can be especially destructive. The goal is to allow participants in the learning network to make rapid adjustments, informing the whole group when they can share what worked in their specific context. A number of robust formative evaluation methods exist that are not at all incompatible with this approach.

- **Facilitation of tacit knowledge exchange:** Many collaboratives go to great lengths to catalogue evidence and build large libraries of general information on how to improve performance. However, as the organizational scientist Ikujiro Nonaka notes, this knowledge can be of limited use. He suggests that practical know-how (or "tacit knowledge"), often contained in the experience of practitioners, generates the most value for others.[10] A well-documented protocol will often pale in comparison to timely advice on how to make that protocol work in a resource-constrained setting or in an environment where staff are resistant. The best collaborative networks will create a lot of space for that kind of informal, just-in-time exchange about the keys to implementation, to the great benefit of their participants.[11]

- **Regular celebration of progress:** Like their colleagues in many professions, healthcare providers rarely experience recognition for their wonderful hard work and creativity. Effective collaborative leaders will address this deficit through proactive celebration of great work and active learning, even when it doesn't immediately lead to improvement. This will give participants additional fuel to persist through the challenges of managing change.

A savvy collaborative leader will track progress on at least some of these dimensions as important proxies for the health of the network and, indeed, as predictors for success at spreading improved outcomes. Moreover, those who fund collaboratives, including foundations and governments, must mindfully create a context for improvement consistent with these operating values. These organizations can, sometimes inadvertently, create an environment of rigidity and fear by requiring excessive adherence to guidelines and inspection at the expense of learning and creativity. In successful cases, however, these funders foster great improvement by encouraging innovation and improvisation, helping all participants meet the collaborative's aims, and introducing expertise and resources on a timely, as-needed basis to further support participants in their shared pursuit of these improvement objectives.

Conclusion

Importantly, effective collaborative leaders will apply similar principles of reflection and learning to themselves and to their work. They will understand that the process of running a collaborative should itself be subject to continuous analysis and improvement. They will energetically seek innovations in running effective collaborative improvement activities and study others across the country and around the world who seek to stimulate large-scale change.

Our hope is that this book helps them on this journey, defining the fundamentals of practice, refining existing skills, and introducing entirely new ideas and approaches to help the field. In addition, we hope that this content provides encouragement and inspiration for this important work, reminding us all of the importance of spreading known, better practice much faster.

Much more than an academic exercise, this activity is chiefly rooted in the belief that we can absolutely reduce the unjust variation in practice that plagues healthcare and deliver to anyone, anywhere, outstanding care.

Everyone has a parent, child, friend or uncle like mine, and they all deserve our very best.

[1] Balas, E., & Boren, S. e. (n.d.). Managing clinical knowledge for health care improvement. Bethesda, Md: National Library of Medicine; 2000. Bemmel J., McCraw A, eds. Yearbook of Medical Informatics.

[2] Fisher, E., Wennberg, D., Stukel, T., & et al. (2003). The implications of regional variations in Medicare spending. Part 1: the content, quality, and accessiblity of care. *Annals of Internal Medicine , 138*, 273-287.

[3] Wennberg, J. (Jan 24, 2005). Variation in use of Medicare services among regions and selected academic medical centers: is more better? *Duncan W. Clark Lecture*. New York Academy of Medicine.

[4] Fisher, E., Goodman, D., Skiiner, J., & Bronner, K. (2009, Feb). Health Care Spending, Quality, and Outcomes. *The Dartmouth Institute for Health Policy and Clinical Practice*.

[5] Gawande, A. (2011, October 3). Personal Best. *New Yorker*.

[6] Rogers, E. (1995). Diffusion of Innovations. *New Yorker: The Free Press*.

[7] Massoud, M., Donohue, K., & McCannon, C. (2010). *Options for Large-Scale Spread of Simple, High-Impact Interventions*. Technical report: USAID Health Care Improvement Project. Bethesda: University Research Co., LLC(URC).

[8] Berwick, D. (2004). Lessons from developing nations on improving health care. *British Medical Journal , 328* (7448), 1124-1129.

[9] Berwick, D. (2004).

[10] Nonaka, I. (1991). The knowledge-creating company. *Harvard Business Review, 69*, 96-104.

[11] Dixon, N. (2000). Common Knowledge. *Harvard Business School Press*.

CHAPTER 2

The Origin and Evolution of the Breakthrough Series Collaborative

By Donald M. Berwick, M.D., MPP
Adapting the Collaborative Model in Africa by Pierre Barker, M.D.

Introduction

Who knows where the expression "two heads are better than one" came from? A British compendium of proverbs says it was first recorded in 1546 in John Heywood's "A dialogue conteinyng the number in effect of all the prouerbes in the Englishe tongue."

"Some heades haue taken two head is better then one: But ten heads without wit, I wene as good none."

The expression gets to the heart of collaboration, which is what this book is all about. Each chapter covers a different aspect of a collaborative.

It's easier to date the beginning of the healthcare collaborative than the "two heads" expressions, too. In fact, I think I was there.

In October 1994, I was sitting next to my friend and colleague, Dr. Paul Batalden, cofounder of the Institute for Healthcare Improvement (IHI). We were at a meeting in Dearborn, Michigan, of the newly formed Group Practice Improvement Network (GPIN). GPIN involved leadership teams from throughout the United States in conferences and activities to help accelerate their care improvement.

Paul and I had often discussed between ourselves and with the IHI Board the stubborn problem of moving from conversation and study, or education for improvement, to action, or engaging informative changes in real care processes "on the ground." For all of the extraordinary success of IHI in the former (IHI courses on quality improvement had long waiting lists and thousands of alumni, for example), we still lacked enough traction on changes in care.

Paul fell silent for a few minutes, scribbling on the back of a paper placemat, and then slid over to me a sketch that has entered the archives of turning points for IHI, and maybe for the healthcare quality movement as a whole (Figure 1).

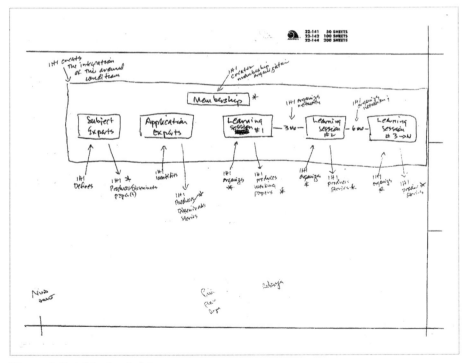

Figure 1. Batalden's sketch

Paul had sketched a way to help organizations band together in what soon became known as a "Breakthrough Series Collaborative." The idea was roughly as follows:

- Pick a topic for improvement as a common focus.
- Engage a panel of experts in that subject-matter field who had achieved better performance than others, or who knew the scientific and engineering foundations for doing so.
- Harvest "change concepts" from those experts.
- Invite care organizations (such as hospitals or group practices) to enroll custom-made teams to join with teams from other organizations in pursuit of that improvement.
- Launch a series of in-person "learning sessions" (Paul drew three on his diagram) at which all of the teams could assemble with the experts; share their approaches, metrics, results, and lessons; and energize periods between the learning sessions ("action periods") with multiple, informative tests of change ("Plan-Do-Study-Act" cycles).
- Use the learning sessions also to teach improvement methods and skills.
- Summarize it all at the end of the project.

Paul's idea struck me as simple, plausible and powerful. I recall redrafting his diagram on the flight back to Boston from GPIN, adding details, if not clarity (Figure 2).

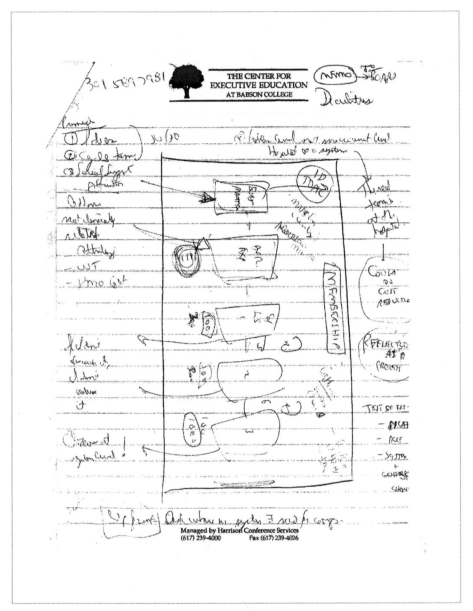

Figure 2. Berwick's embellished version of Batalden's sketch

I'm amused to notice today that the upper-left corner of my diagram includes a telephone number—it's the number of Tom Nolan, Ph.D., a statistician and protégé of W. Edwards Deming, who had become a close friend and key advisor to IHI and to me. Tom, perhaps more than any other single individual, provided (and continues to provide) intellectual leadership for much of the progress of IHI through the years. He had several times commented to me and other IHI leaders that the quality movement wouldn't last long if it stayed focused on training, rather than action. I called him to seek reactions and guidance on the idea of collaborative improvement. He liked it.

The Breakthrough Series and Open Access Models are Born

My ride home from Detroit was not comfortable, because although I could see the power of Dr. Batalden's template, I couldn't see how to translate the model into an actual IHI program. Luckily, Penny Carver was at IHI, and I handed the drafts to her and asked to see what could be made of them. Within a few days and after a few more iterations, the Breakthrough Series (Figure 3) was born.

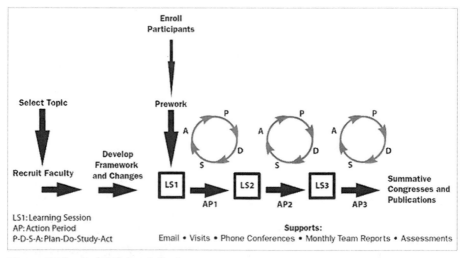

Figure 3. The Breakthrough Series

Penny developed the proper mechanics of faculty recruitment, organizational invitation, meeting planning and whatever else it took to make the project a reality. The next step was to select the topics IHI would focus on, and that became the job of the senior leaders and senior faculty of IHI, who, in short order, generated criteria and a first list.

The criteria were more or less obvious: For example, pick topics of clinical importance to patients and (when possible) financial importance to organizations. Ensure that experts (either academics, or practitioners or both) could likely be found who know how to achieve much better performance than usual. And try to choose cycle times and scale that permitted noticeable improvement within a few weeks or months—as opposed to years. For the experts, IHI could exploit its already vast network of faculty and organizations, seeing best practice sites and great ideas for change.

The first topic chosen was Caesarean section rates. They had crept to more than 30 percent in many places in the U.S., and the American College of Obstetrics and Gynecology had recommended rates closer to 15 percent. Dr. Bruce Flamm at Kaiser Permanente was a well-published clinical leader offering ideas about how to achieve lower rates safely. He was recruited to become the first-ever chair of an IHI Breakthrough Series project, Reducing C-Section Rates Safely, which was launched in May of 1995, with 28 participating organizations.

The initial package of ideas included 11 "change concepts" for the teams. The project lasted about two years, and the results were reported in the journal, Birth, in 1995.[1] Of 28 participating organizations, 15 percent reduced cesarean delivery rates by 30 percent or more during the 12-month period of active collaborative work. An additional 50 percent reduced them between 10 and 30 percent.

That first collaborative project ushered in a steady stream of IHI Breakthrough Series projects. Between 1995 and 2005, IHI organized and led 52 Breakthrough Series Collaboratives on 35 different improvement topics, including Reducing Waits and Delays, Improving Outcomes in Cardiac Surgery, Improving Care at the End of Life, and many more. Typical collaboratives had between 30 and 60 organizational members and teams, but IHI began pushing the envelope with collaboratives of a much larger size.[2]

A turning point on scale came when then-Undersecretary for Health of the Veterans' Health Administration Dr. Ken Kizer got wind of the success IHI was realizing with a series of collaboratives to reduce waits and delays in healthcare. Under the intellectual leadership of a Kaiser Permanente physician named Mark Murray, teams in prior IHI collaboratives were applying and adapting basic change concepts derived from queuing theory to reduce waits and delays dramatically with no increases in staff or space, and with unprecedented levels of access for patients in what became known as the Open Access model. Open Access essentially gave patients the ability to name the time and date of their visits, including same-day options, while reducing the burden on staff and clinicians.

In 1999, Dr. Kizer asked IHI to bring Open Access and the Breakthrough Series model to the Veterans Health Administration, but he wasn't interested in a stepwise deployment. He insisted that all of the 22 Vertically Integrated Service Networks (VISNs), with a total of 134 VA centers, be engaged in one collaborative from the start. IHI took the bait, and the momentum and results were impressive.

For example, in the first project, which engaged participating clinics from all VISNs from July 1999, to March 2000 median waiting times for visits in primary care and specialty clinics fell 54 percent, from 48 days to 22 days. The project continued and expanded over the next two years, and waiting times for primary care appointments throughout the VA fell from more than 60.4 days to 28.4 days. VISN 2, which was actively using the collaborative approach throughout its sites, achieved waiting times of 16 days.[3] This extraordinary progress using the Breakthrough Series as a learning model shows how a managed system organized to learn can make achievements at scale, and makes the recent access problems in the VA all the more poignant given that system's demonstrated potential for large-scale improvement.

It was around that time, the late 1990s, when another giant step for collaborative improvement models took shape, this time in England. The new Labour Party Government of Prime Minister Tony Blair was well aware of public discontent with poor access and long waiting times in the English National Health Service (NHS), and they felt a political imperative to reduce waits, among other NHS reforms. Early in Blair's first term of office, the Government established a Modernisation Board (on which I served) and, based on its recommendations, a new "Modernisation Agency" (MA) for the NHS. The MA was to oversee and facilitate widespread improvements of care according to priorities established by the NHS, the foremost of which was to reduce waits and delays.

Two years before the MA was created, Dr. John Oldham, a British general practitioner from Derbyshire, who had established a reputation for sound clinical management and innovation, had already set up the Primary Care Development Team (PCDT) to work nationally on waiting times and coronary heart disease management. Dr. Oldham had mastered and further developed both the Open Access model (which he called Advanced Access) and the Breakthrough Series model, which he had learned from IHI.

Over two years, Dr. Oldham learned to operate waves of interlinked collaboratives in a hub-and-spoke model. This brought collaboratives to a scale never before seen anywhere, for example eventually leading a network of 11 regional PCDT organizations—a nodal architecture—and reducing waiting times dramatically for more than 32 million Britains, and earning Dr. Oldham a knighthood in the process.[4,5]

The MA built on and expanded such collaborative work to a wide range of clinical and administrative processes.

As IHI continued to roll out one Breakthrough Series collaborative after another, large, multihospital systems and integrated delivery systems began to adopt and adapt the method for internal use coordinating the improvement efforts of their component entities.

For example, Dr. David Pryor and his colleagues used collaboratives within the Ascension Health system of hospitals to accelerate progress on patient safety. The Bureau of Primary Care in the Health Resources and Services Administration undertook with IHI a massive collaborative on chronic illness care improvement in nearly 800 community health centers. The Indian Health Service began a similar effort on chronic illness and prevention. In the state of Michigan, with help from Johns Hopkins University, the Keystone Patient Safety project, launched in 2003, involved more than 100 intensive care units in efforts to reduce ICU infections, with remarkable results.[6]

To support this replication and spread of collaborative improvement, in 2001 IHI launched the Breakthrough Series College. This has been offered 25 times since and has trained more than 1,400 leaders to date in various approaches to forming and managing such projects.

A number of national healthcare programs in other countries began to exploit collaborative approaches. This included, for example, patient safety programs in Scotland, Wales, Denmark, Japan and Sweden. As of this writing that trend continues, with national projects starting in 2015, for example in Portugal to improve patient safety and in Brazil to reduce Caesarean-section rates.

Perhaps most interesting have been the applications of the collaborative model in developing countries. Dr. Pierre Barker and his global health team at IHI, for example, led successful projects with governments in South Africa on HIV-AIDS care, in Malawi on maternal and neonatal mortality, and Ghana on mortality in children under 5 years of age.[7,8,9]

Dr. M. Rashad Massoud and his team at URC, building on Sir John Oldham's pioneering nodal designs, developed an expanded model for collaboratives using a "wave" structure of serial projects and using "champions" from prior waves to assist the next waves in developing nations to reach enormous scale rapidly.[10,11]

Dr. Barker's and Dr. Massoud's groups, in essence, adapted the Breakthrough Series model to new organizational, political, economic and cultural contexts, especially in resource-poor settings. They learned how to make modifications such as using coaches, regional meetings, and cell phone technologies where geography and financial constraints made large, face-to-face meetings especially difficult. Dr. Barker offers his commentary on the richness of adaptation of the original collaborative structure to the African context (see sidebar).

As administrator of the Centers for Medicare and Medicaid Services from July 2010, to December 2011, I had the chance to launch the Partnership for Patients with resources from the CMS Center for Medicare and Medicaid Innovation (CMMI), created by the Affordable Care Act. The Partnership for Patients included at its core collaborative learning structures and supports, implemented largely through a series of Hospital Engagement Networks. Its results

Adapting the Collaborative Model in Africa
By Pierre Barker M.D.

The Breakthrough Series model has proven highly applicable to efforts to improve performance of the more centrally directed, district-based health systems in Africa. The adaptation of the model to these settings led to a number of innovations that may have a wider application in better-resourced environments such as the U.S. health system. The lack of Internet connectivity necessitated more reliance on change agents who pollinated change ideas across sites in the network through multiple visits. Because the "change packages" had not been assembled or tested previously in Africa, the Breakthrough Series model, initially developed in the U.S. as a mechanism to foster adoption and spread, became a learning system that was used primarily for innovation of changes that could then be spread.

The model was also used as a spread mechanism for IHI's Ghana project on maternal and neonatal mortality, but the challenges encountered in logistics and resources required for national scale-up in these settings suggests that other spread mechanisms (e.g., campaign used in 100,000 Lives) may be more efficient approaches to large-scale spread. In South Africa, the Breakthrough Series was used for innovating and demonstrating effective implementation of HIV care at a district level, and developing change packages that were then spread throughout the national healthcare system using a more centrally directed approach."[12]

are still under study, but significant improvements in rates of hospital-acquired conditions and readmissions seem well in hand.

So, the collaborative model that Dr. Batalden sketched on a placemat in 1994 has in the 21 years since become a mainstay of improvement efforts worldwide for organizations, multi-organizational system, regions and nations. It has changed with time and with the good thinking and lessons learned from adopters everywhere.

Indeed, today some of its forms look very different from that first project on C-section rates. The Keystone program emphasized standardized metrics and independent assessments. The URC model added a highly structured series of waves for spread. And many sponsors, including IHI, have exploited web-based virtual exchanges to supplement and even replace face-to-face meetings.

Common Questions About the Breakthrough Series Model

Like many innovations—especially social change innovations—collaborative improvement methods in general and the IHI Breakthrough Series model in particular have had their share of skeptical critics. Questions raised, some repeatedly, include these, for example:

- **Doubts about the scientific discipline of measurement, inference and results reporting:** Many collaborative projects have been undertaken in settings and under circumstances in which classical forms of experimental control, especially randomization, can't or shouldn't be used. Evaluations depend more upon pre-post comparisons and time-series analyses, which some find insufficiently convincing.
- **Doubts about the data:** Collaboratives rely largely upon self-reported data, rather than independent outside inspection. (In truth, a number of IHI-sponsored

collaboratives have been the subjects of serious outside evaluation.) Critics question the validity, objectivity and reliability of self-reported data. On the other hand, as Dr. Oldham has pointed out, very few, if any, classical experimental studies have the volume of data and participants that collaboratives do. The large amount of data coupled with the use of measurement over time give collaboratives statistical power that's rare in formal experimental designs.

- **Doubts about attribution:** Collaboratives do their work in the messy, real world of continually changing context and intersections efforts. The world doesn't stand still, holding its breath for a collaborative to be completed. Rules change; knowledge changes; parallel improvement efforts come and go. Purists who seek certainty in attribution—that "A" caused "B"—will be unsatisfied by the processes of inference upon which the evaluation of social changes must rely. Furthermore, most collaboratives don't rely on single interventions. Instead, they often teach and test packages of interventions that IHI calls "change packages," in which teasing out the effect of each component isn't at all the primary agenda. If the bundle of changes helps, that's progress, whether or not we're crystal clear about the contribution of each element of the bundle.

- **Doubts about sustainability:** The original IHI Breakthrough Series model contemplated projects of specific duration—18 or 24 months, for example. Even if apparently successful, do these results last for the long haul?

In addition, both the collaborative model and the subject-matter changes they support on specific topics tend to be unstable. They change over time—happily so, in my view. With respect to the conduct of collaboratives, smart people keep trying new ways to support shared improvement. Are face-to-face meetings, which are costly, truly needed? How many? Should metrics be standardized? To what degree? What rhythm of reporting from participants helps? How can we best exploit the web and virtual connectivity? What about physical visits among participants?

It's important to acknowledge, just as Dr. Barker does in the African context, that as powerful as collaboratives are now proven to be in their numerous forms, it's not a panacea nor is it a necessary or sufficient approach under all circumstances. In the time since the Breakthrough Series first appeared, other approaches to large-scale spread of change have also developed in (or been adapted to) healthcare, such as campaigns, extension agents and social mobilization movements, to name just a few.[13] Much has yet to be learned about where collaboratives reach the limits of their effectiveness in duration, size and topic area. The important attention now being given in healthcare to truly transformational redesigns of care and approaches to improving population health may stretch collaborative designs beyond their capacity (or maybe not).

Beyond any doubt, the movement toward collaborative improvement is a dynamic one, with growth and development rather than fixed forms. It's for that reason, primarily, that the seductive question, "Do collaboratives work?" has no crisp answer and never will, any more than there's a single answer to the question, "Does parenting work?" or "Does schooling work?"

As the originator of the Breakthrough Series model, Dr. Batalden says, "The idea (of collaborative improvement) is better seen as a learning strategy— an action learning strategy—not as an intervention that should be evaluated as a new treatment should be."[14]

The more appropriate approaches to helping collaboratives get better are well explored among the developers and practitioners of "realistic evaluation" and other forms of inquiry appropriately sensitive to details of contexts and mechanisms.[15] But, unhappily, evaluators of collaboratives too often fail to consider these approaches and the underlying epistemological challenges.

Conclusion

Despite the questions, controversies, skeptics and limitations, collaboratives continue to spread, evolve and thrive, now on a global basis. To realize why, one only has to become involved with one. In a healthcare landscape afflicted in all countries by economic and social pressures, regulatory demands and forces of surveillance, the morale of health care workers in all roles is at risk. It's just the opposite in the heart of a well-managed collaborative, marked by an ethos of mutual respect, teamwork, optimism, the joy of learning and the focus on purpose.

Most important, as IHI Senior Vice President Dr. Kedar Mate put it, "The bedrock value within a collaborative is freedom from fear in any form—fear of inspection, fear of failure, fear of reprisal."[16]

Coupling freedom from fear with other values like inclusiveness, respect, a bias toward action and the embrace of reflection, collaboratives create a space for learning and progress that seems all too rare in traditional corporate environments.

Sometimes the results are thrilling, often the results are simply affirming, but almost always the sense of empowerment, openness and engagement feeds the spirit of people who have decided that working together to improve beats loneliness every time.

---

[1] Flamm BL, Berwick DM, Kabcenell A. Reducing cesarean section rates safely: lessons from a "breakthrough series" collaborative. Birth 1998, 25: 117-24.

[2] *The Breakthrough Series: IHI's Collaborative Model for Achieving Breakthrough Improvement.* IHI Innovation Series white paper. Boston: Institute for Healthcare Improvement; 2003. (Available on www.IHI.org) (http://www.ihi.org/resources/Pages/IHIWhitePapers/TheBreakthrough SeriesIHIsCollaborativeModel forAchievingBreakthroughImprovement.aspx)

[3] Nolan K, Schall MW, Erb F, Nolan T. Using a framework for spread: the case of patient access in the Veterans Health Administration. Joint Comm J Qual Patient Safety. 2005; 31:339-47.

[4] Oldham J. *Sic Evenit Ratio ut componitur* (the small book about large system change). London: Kingsham Press, 2004 ISBN 1-904235-27-1.

[5] Oldham J. JAMA. 2009; Achieving large system change in healthcare. JAMA 2009; 301:965-6.

[6] Pronovost P, Needham D, Berenholtz S, et al. An intervention to decrease catheter-related bloodstream infections in the ICU. N Engl J Med. 2006;355:2725-2732.

[7] Webster PD, Sibanyoni M, Malekutu D, Mate KS, Venter WD, Barker PM, Moleko W. Using quality improvement to accelerate highly active antiretroviral treatment coverage in South Africa. BMJ Qual Saf. 2012 Apr;21(4):315-24.

[8] Mate KS, Ngubane G, Barker PM. A quality improvement model for the rapid scale-up of a program to prevent mother-to-child HIV transmission in South Africa. Int J Qual Health Care. 2013 Sep;25(4):373-80.

[9] Twum-Danso NA, Akanlu GB, Osafo E, Sodzi-Tettey S, Boadu RO, Atinbire S, Adondiwo A, Amenga-Etego I, Ashagbley F, Boadu EA, Dasoberi I, Kanyoke E, Yabang E, Essegbey IT, Adjei GA, Buckle GB, Awoonor-Williams JK, Nang-Beifubah A, Twumasi A, McCannon CJ, Barker PM. A nationwide quality improvement project to accelerate Ghana's progress toward Millennium Development Goal Four: design and implementation processes. Int J Qual Health Care. 2012 Dec;24(6):601-1.

[10] Massoud MR, Mensah-Abrampah N. A promising approach to scale up health care improvements in low- and middle-income countries: The Wave Sequence Spread Approach and the concept of the Slice of the System. 2014; F1000 Research; 3:100.

[11] Massoud MR, Mensah-Abrampah N. Scaling Up of High Impact Interventions. In, Beracochea E (ed). Improving Aid Effectiveness in Global Health. Springer, 2015.

[12] Barker P. Personal communication. Email of August 22, 2015.

[13] Massoud MR, Donohue K, McCannon CJ. Options for Large-Scale Spread of Simple, High-Impact Interventions. *Technical Report*. Published by USAID Health Care Improvement Project. Bethesda, MD: University Research Co., LLC (URC). (Joint publication of USAID, World Health Organization, Harvard School of Public Health, Institute for Healthcare Improvement.) 2010.

[14] Batalden P. Personal communication. Email of August 17, 2015.

[15] Pawson R, Tilley N. Realistic Evaluation. (London: Sage Publications, Ltd; 1997.)

[16] Mate K. Personal communication. Email of August 19, 2015.

CHAPTER 3

Adopting Innovation and Change Management

By Jeff Thompson, M.D. and Patricia A. Teske, RN, MHA

Introduction

I was on a call with a professor from University of Southern California who described the need for both a top-down and bottom-up approach to improve safety and resiliency in highly complex organizations such as healthcare. He said it's like planting a seed. You need to have a strong seed, dig the hole and prepare the soil while attending to conditions in the environment such as water and light. Leaving any of these out will result in a plant that doesn't grow or thrive.

This simple metaphor resonated with me. When using a collaborative to spread lasting changes in healthcare, we need to attend to the collaborative, the actual innovation and the organizations we're asking to adopt the innovation. If we have an ineffective collaborative, an insignificant innovation or an unprepared organization, we're unlikely to reach our collaborative aim.

Subsequent chapters will detail the elements of an effective collaborative and describe thinking around selecting interventions. In this chapter we'll explore factors associated with adopting innovation at the organizational level, and address human behavior and decision-making that will help lead change efforts. We're fortunate to have many outstanding healthcare leaders contribute to this book. One such leader is Dr. Jeff Thompson, retired CEO of Gundersen Health System. Jeff offered to describe the way his organization prepared to be an effective collaborative participant with the ability to adapt and adopt innovations. Here's what he has to say.

Structure Leads to Innovation

If you want innovation, provide structure. This isn't conventional wisdom, but the highest performers still want to know where the fences are and what the overall goals are. In the next few pages we'll describe ways to provide an appropriate amount and type of structure to deliver increasing creativity and innovation.

First, clarity around the organization's goals and its strategic plan must be thoughtful and consistent. It needs to be used to provide a template for planning, decision-making and individual actions. It's equally important to have a model that gives people a path forward for behavior. For example, a compact (not a contract) that clearly explains what's going to be delivered by the organization and what's going to be delivered by the individual sets a tone of mutual responsibility and transparency.

Next, if you only give staff clear goals without great tools you provide a perfect environment for anxiety. It's important to provide consistent information across all team members and an improvement system that makes sense and is workable, as well as improvement training that serves the strategic plan and supports behaviors consistent with the compact. It's equally important to develop the discipline of allowing changes.

With this approach, people know what's expected of the organization; where the organization is going; what's expected of them personally; what tools they will have; and how progress will be measured, evaluated and improved. It will feel like a predictable rhythm in a fair, thoughtful system.

Similarly, thoughtful strategic planning, a participation commitment and other necessary tools must be in place at the collaborative level. Organizations want to participate in collaboratives that work on topics of strategic importance to them. They want to know what they'll get and what they need to give before they commit to participate. Having a clear aim at the start will establish the goal for what the collaborative wants its participating organizations to accomplish and when this goal will be reached. Collaboratives need to have or facilitate the sharing of effective ideas and tools to support the adaptation and adoption of innovation at the organizational level.

Gundersen Health System's Strategic Plan

Let's discuss an example: Gundersen Health System's strategic plan. The plan is structured around three-, five- and 10-year scenarios and begins with a short, crisp **purpose statement:** *Our purpose is to bring health and well-being to our patients and communities.* Even the most casual reader instantly sees that the organization's interest is greater than just a sick patient showing up at a hospital or clinic. It's about health and well-being, which includes physical health as well as mental, social and financial health of patients and the community. So a purpose statement can set a tone and an understanding that helps organize thinking across the organization. How does this help the individual? It lets them know where the broad boundaries are and what the priorities will be in the organization. They can build within the organization, or start developing pathways, for partnership and collaboration outside the traditional lines.

The **mission** is clear: *We will distinguish ourselves through excellence in patient care, education, research and improved health in the communities we serve.* The organization will excel, not just exist, and its mission goal is clear. So if you get through the top two lines on purpose and mission, you already know the aim is to increase the well-being of the community. More specifically, you're not aiming for mediocrity, but excellence. A staff member can see how broad and high the playing field is.

The **vision statement** defines the goal: *We will be a health system of excellence, nationally recognized for improving the health and well-being of our patients, families and their communities.* It provides clarity about what we're going to measure against: We'll be so good we'll be nationally recognized. This will embolden innovators saying they want to push, to take on the best. You can only know if you're better by measuring, comparing and interacting with the best.

A **commitment statement** is added more for operations than innovation: *We will deliver high-quality care because lives depend on it, service as though the patient were a loved one, and relentless improvement because our future depends on it.* It's there to let people who may not identify with national recognition understand how their work saves lives and connects with a loved one. It also adds clarity about why we need to get better and supports the drive of innovators by saying our whole future depends on it. This section sets the tone of serving something bigger than yourself, aiming to be as good as anyone, and providing a framework so an innovator knows how broad the field is and how high the goals can be set. A criticism of this approach is that it may put off frontline employees who say they can't have that huge of an impact, but that will be dealt with later in the methodology of improvement.

The **values section** gives people a roadmap for behavior:

- *Integrity: Perform with honesty, responsibility and transparency*
- *Excellence: Measure and achieve excellence in all aspects of delivering healthcare*
- *Respect: Treat patients, families and coworkers with dignity*
- *Innovation: Embrace change and contribute new ideas*
- *Compassion: Provide compassionate care to patients and families*

These items will carry you to success. Once again, high-performing individuals want to know what's expected of them, where the fences are, and how they're going to get along in the chosen environment. Innovation is called out, but the truth is that an environment with respect, integrity and excellence are as important to supporting innovative staff as calling out the value of innovation itself.

The strategic plan finishes with five major strategies around quality and safety, patient experience, culture, affordability and growth. While it's not terribly unique in healthcare to have strategies that lead with quality, safety and service, this plan is exceptional because the strategies take the tone of caregiver and emphasize that patients should provide input into deciding what success looks like. For example, under the patient experience strategy one bullet reads: **Partner with patients and families to design and deliver their ideal care experience.**

Finally, there's **growth.** Innovators love to see the term growth, but we narrow it down. We don't say growth for growth's sake, or growth just to get bigger, or growth to say that we're bigger. We have **growth as a tool**, or as a way to serve the rest of the organization, the patients and the communities. We have different ways of connecting with different partners. Although there's a great deal of structure in the mission, vision, value and strategic plan, it offers many opportunities to unleash the creativity of the staff.

Collaboratives differ in their structures. Some organize around a topic and disband, while others are more perpetual networks that continue on with new topics when they're finished with one. While many collaboratives don't compose a purpose statement, mission, vision statement and commitment statement, at least in the way a traditional organization might, they all have some specific aim that describes what they want to accomplish and the timeframe. Those designing and running collaboratives should ask themselves: Are the goals of my collaborative in alignment with the strategic plans for the organizations I wish to recruit?

Sometimes a collaborative may be on the leading edge of change that hasn't yet been considered or prioritized by the organizations it wishes to recruit.

If this is the case the collaborative should consider strategies appropriate to the pre-contemplation stage described by Prochaska's Stages of Change Model[1]. Provide education about the change and the expected benefit to the organization, explore potential concerns and keep the door open for further consideration. Collaborative leaders should be aware of the social psychology associated with change and use strategies aligned with the organization's level of readiness[2]. For example, the collaborative could leverage the social psychology of change by appealing to the organization's desire to be part of something bigger than themselves, joining a cause that's important nationally or that their peers have already committed to.

Setting Expectations

Clarifying behavior expectations among staff is another key component for innovation and creativity. After years of managing the medical staff, which is critical to the health and well-being of a health system, we decided to codify that behavior in writing. We started with the medical staff since they're often pointed out as the biggest problem and the biggest opportunity. If they set the appropriate tone, there's a better chance of that tone persisting.

We developed a medical staff compact that started with our organizational values practiced by the CEO and medical vice presidents. Young members of the medical staff who were in leadership training edited the document, which lists Gundersen Health System's Responsibilities alongside the Medical Staff's Responsibilities.

This particular tool has proved invaluable because it clearly outlines what the organization will deliver to a medical staff member and what a medical staff member will deliver to the organization. It's open, transparent and in writing: If we fail to deliver they can hold it up and say, "Here's your promise, you're falling short." Likewise, before a physician fills out an application and signs an employment agreement, he or she has the opportunity to consider and discuss the expectations.

For example, applicants have occasionally been put off by a "treat everyone with respect" line under Medical Staff's Responsibilities. But as a disciplined organization we can't waiver on these expectations regardless of the short-term potential implications for the organization or singular department. This is not without pain and there are struggles. But making sure all medical staff members behave in a fashion consistent with the compact sets the same bar as the administrative leads and now the compact spreads to the rest of the organization. Again, this is not a contract but a clarity of understanding: Here's what's expected of the organization and you. This creates an environment where people can spend their energy on improvement, innovation and development rather than wasting energy battling bad behaviors and interpersonal interactions. These expectations are also part of all staff evaluations.

For those designing and running collaboratives, the question to ask is: Are the commitments expected of the collaborative and for the participants clear? When designing and running a collaborative there can be a tension between having a very low bar for participation in order to bring more organizations into the effort vs. setting higher expectations for participants to weed out those not truly dedicated to making necessary changes. Regardless of the expectations you have for commitment they should be clearly communicated to potential participants to the fullest extent possible during the recruitment phase. If circumstances change over the course of the collaborative it's important to quickly and transparently share any changes in expectations with the participating organizations. This topic is discussed more fully in chapter 7 on recruiting and optimizing participants.

It's also important to anticipate the impact of the new innovation on the organization. Collaboratives should help their organizational partners make the right thing to do the easy thing to do. This approach has been key to many successes, such as developing central line insertion trays that contain all of the supplies needed to perform the insertion using proper technique. Collaboratives and organizations should anticipate that it will be easier to make changes that impact a smaller, more cohesive patient populations such as implementing the ventilator associated pneumonia bundle than it is to reduce all-cause readmissions. Some change efforts have a clearly defined evidence base while others have a set of ideas that need to be tested and aligned with the individual needs of the organization.

If new behaviors don't become the norm despite setting clear expectations and providing training and peer support, collaborative and organizational leaders should explore why rather than setting mandates or punishment for non-compliance. Do practitioners have a fear of the unknown? Does the change create a loss for the practitioner in status, autonomy or connection? Create an environment where feedback and testing are encouraged. The new way may not be a better way and may need to be adapted to work within the organization.

So clarity of expectations, high goals and guidelines for behavior all make sense, but only work if staff members have the tools to accomplish those things. Setting goals and timelines is easy; managing the anxiety of an unsupported staff takes a lot of time and is very inefficient. Our approach has been to develop a very broad educational program that includes onsite electronic educational activities for frontline staff, managers, directors, medical staff leads and executive education pathways that have the potential to become the CEO.

The Education Framework

Like most organizations we have an extensive online educational framework. Ours, called GundU, has a vast array of both required and optional education for all staff in the organization. We think this is necessary, but just a baseline. To really drive creativity and problem-solving and stimulate innovation among the breadth of the staff, you need a strong leadership education focus. With well-trained medical and administrative leads who are open to improvement, it's more likely that inspired staff will find fertile ground as they push us forward.

We have a framework for all leadership. Our philosophy for physician leadership development is that physicians have inherent leadership skills, and we enhance them by providing the business skills necessary to deliver on our mission. We develop leadership job charters from the organization's strategic vision to use in hiring and selecting leaders. We craft their individual development and consistently evaluate their performance and that of the organization. We use performance reviews and individual development reviews to form a learning plan that's consistent with both current performance and future development needs of the individual (Figure 1). There are multiple layers for multiple roles within the organization.

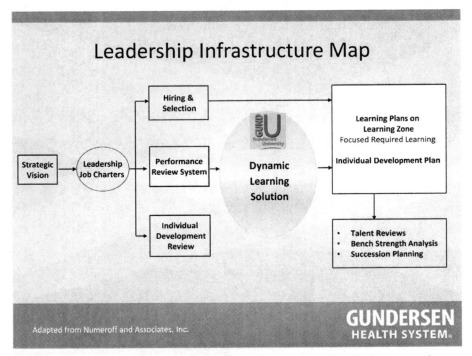

Figure 1. Hiring and selecting leaders is based on leadership job charters and learning plans are based on performance and development reviews.

For early career, we have leadership book groups available for all members of the provider and administrative parts of the organization, and a one- to two-year Learning Community for new physician leaders. For mid-career, there are a number of internal activities, including department chair college, courses on our online education framework, GundU, and individual communication and service coaching. External education and training are also available and supported in the organization.

Not all those introduced to leadership will choose to move forward, and not all those who choose to move forward will do well. A great organization will provide individuals with clarity on what it takes to lead, the tools to help them rise up to leadership, and honesty in evaluating and guiding them along their paths.

So now we have goals, behavior expectations and educational activity. We also need consistency in the improvement and education approach among different groups, such as managers, directors and medical staff leads.

Ensuring Consistency

We developed the Gundersen Improvement System that we teach in an attempt to extract innovation from all parts of the organization (Figure 2). We use a change acceleration process (CAP) created by General Electric because of its ability to develop a shared need and get engagement from frontline staff. Staff need to feel connected and excited about how this is important to them and their patients, so developing that shared need is critical.

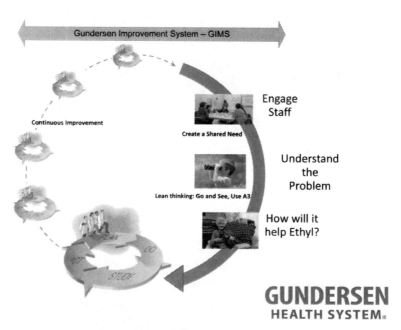

Figure 2. Gundersen Improvement System helps to lead and manage change.

We also believe that lean methodology, creating more value with fewer resources, is one of the most useful tools in healthcare. The lean management and improvement system and its A3 (named after the size of a piece of paper) problem-solving process have been an important part of our innovative success[3]. When you develop a shared need and use the CAP process of shaping a vision, mobilizing commitment, making change last and monitoring progress, you change systems and structures. Using the A3 tool, anyone on the frontline can answer the question, "What's going on now?" to determine the current state. This enables most staff to easily see the best future state. Since they live the work, they can develop an expansive list of barriers, obstacles and opportunities to improve.

Dr. John Toussaint, CEO of ThedaCare Center for Healthcare Value, a lean education institute for healthcare change, said he wishes the approach was not called lean or A3 in reference to healthcare, but "scientific method of process improvement." Many clinicians have balked at the idea of fixing people the way lean manufacturing fixes cars. However, the lean methodology is as adaptable to healthcare as it is to manufacturing. The advantage is that front-line staff can be engaged, and large or small systems can be evaluated, and this flows into the Plan-Do-Study-Act (PDSA) cycle, a trial-and-learning method for testing changes, made popular by the Institute for Healthcare Improvement (IHI). This very simple approach at the frontlines, with just a couple tools, gives legs to what otherwise could be a frustrating situation. These tools embedded in a clear management system gives the staff a clear path forward and reduces the anxiety and pressure of the need for constant change and improvement.

If you're designing and running a collaborative, ask yourself the following questions:

- Have you planned adequate knowledge exchange to support the organizations within your collaborative?

- Does your education plan include topic-specific content and information on developing and strengthening leadership skills?
- Do you have subject-matter experts, and have you identified local clinical champions? Ideally, clinical champions are opinion leaders, either formal or informal, who are regarded for their judgment and outcomes. Champions can use new behaviors and encourage their peers to test them as well. Champions can call out peers who are not behaving appropriately. Champions may self-identify or can be identified by others when they are asked, "Who would you go to if....?"
- Does your knowledge exchange provide guidelines for the organization that go beyond clinical intervention?
- Are teams taught to work with the most interested and engaged people first, rather than attempting to convert the laggards?
- Are teams taught to look for bright spots within their organization, where the desired process is working well, so they can learn why it's working and spread the effective concepts elsewhere in the organization?
- Do the participating organizations use a specific performance-improvement methodology or their own selection? Do you require participants to use the same methodology?
- Do you need to provide technical support for organizations to help them increase their quality-improvement capacity?
- Do you provide the opportunity for group discussion and discovery?
- Do you have a system in place to provide feedback to your participating organizations and to learn from them about the barriers they may be facing as well as their successes?

Discipline

Again, it doesn't seem logical that discipline and innovation should go together; but when we talk about discipline, it's what Jim Collins describes in his book "Good to Great."[4] It has nothing to do with pulling out bad apples and standing them in the corner; but it has everything to do with a thoughtful, organized approach where staff members understand what's expected of them and there's predictable follow-through. People who are hardworking innovators are happy to get measured. They want to know what the measures are going to be; they want to know what they have to get done by when; and they're quite willing to provide performance to meet those requirements.

Our approach was to record performance electronically early on, so it's immediately available across the organization. Every manager, every director, as they turn on their computers each day, can get a full screen of the various measures on each part of their strategic plan. This allows them to adjust, to inquire, to fix the issues if they're not right, and to fix the processes if the outcomes aren't right in real time. It doesn't always work that easy. Sometimes when the outcomes look bad, the response is to say that the data is bad. You have to prove that the numbers are sound and not fall into the trap of saying "we're a special case" or "our patients are sicker" (this is probably one of the most common in healthcare).

To address this and help move along our innovation more quickly, Gundersen helped form a consortium of healthcare providers across Wisconsin that agrees to develop common definitions and report outcomes to a common source so they can compare to each other, learn who is the best and learn from them.

One of the great joys in healthcare is that people with better outcomes are almost always quite willing to share them with others, including competitors (http://www.wchq.org/). When common excuses are taken away, it sets the stage for a more forward-focused, creative approach to problem-solving.

What really helps drive improvement is the combination of making sure the data you're responsible for is good enough, making comparisons against the external world, and defending your performance on a regular rhythm. This is the reporting cycle in our organization, where twice a year the department chair, who is a physician, and the administrative director, who is a non-physician, report on their results. They report on Gundersen's strategies of quality, patient experience, workplace culture, affordability and growth. They focus on where they've succeeded in their goals, and where they've failed, but mostly on what their next plans are.

What will they change? How will they change? What new approaches will they take? This encourages innovation in the midst of this otherwise disciplined approach. They present this to the senior vice presidents and the CEO. It's a chance for staff to demonstrate their capabilities, and for senior staff to help understand who they need to help, who they need to promote and who may need a different type of opportunity. It's a catalyst that, when taken back to the front line, A3s or PDSAs, it boosts the energy for change and improvement.

Gundersen's structured environment may seem like an unlikely place for innovation. But within it, the most effective advanced-care planning program in the world was generated and spread across multiple countries. The most effective environmental sustainability program was developed and is now showing places across the United States how to move forward. A long-term comprehensive weight-management program that includes portion control, and classes and broad community engagement was developed in this structured environment long before our best-of-class surgery.

Multiple clinical innovations, including minimally invasive cardiac surgery and leading breast cancer care, have all come out of an environment that on paper might look too structured. In reality, it frees up individuals to expand their thinking and serve their communities on an ever-increasing, broader stage. We would argue that the structure around who we are and where we're going, what our priorities are, how we're going to treat each other, and how we're going to treat our communities provides a great opportunity for innovation.

Persistence and discipline at an individual organization will serve a collaborative as well. For those designing and running a collaborative, ask yourself the following questions:

- What's the system and cycle for feedback and action planning within your collaborative?
- Are periodic check-ins with improvement teams and organizational leaders scheduled and structured?
- Are follow-up activities tracked?

For a seed to grow and a plant to thrive, we need a strong seed, fertile planting and positive environmental conditions. Assuming that a collaborative has valuable innovation worth spreading, it will likely be more successful when it partners with organizations that have the ability to receive, adapt and implement the innovation. The keys are alignment with participating organizations' strategic goals; clearly established expectations for participation, training and communication with an eye toward leadership and capacity building at the organization's level; and the discipline of participants to continuously learn and provide feedback and support.

A collaborative is a marathon, not a sprint, and adaptation and persistence are necessary characteristics.

[1] Prochaska, J. O., & DiClemente, C. C. (1983). Stages and processes of self-change of smoking: Toward an integrative model of change. *Journal of Consulting and Clinical Psychology, 51* (3), 390.

[2] Prochaska, J. O., DiClemente, C. C., & Norcross, J. C. (1992). In search of how people change: Applications to addictve behaviors. *American Psychologist, 47* (9), 1102-1114.

[3] Brandao de Souza, L. (2009). Trends and approaches in lean healthcare. *Leadership in Health Services , 2* (2), 121-139.

[4] Collins, J. (2001). *Good to Great: Why Some Companies Make The Leap...And Others Don't.* New York, New York: HarperCollins Publisher, Inc.

CHAPTER 4

The Key Elements of Effective Collaborative Design—Fostering Leadership at All Levels

By Dennis Wagner, MPA, Dan Buffington, Pharm.D., MBA, John Scanlon, Ph.D. and Paul McGann, M.D.

Introduction

Every effective collaborative we've encountered was successful because the participating individuals chose to make something happen that was important and out of the ordinary. This kind of choice is a leadership act. These people had a leadership vision of a compelling future and they stepped forward to align it with the collaborative aim.

In many cases it was the collaborative process that helped individuals recognize what they stood for and gave them opportunities to act on it. Collaboratives can be made more powerful by cultivating and calling on the leadership qualities inherent in each of us. Leadership grows and spreads with recognition.

This chapter includes practical experiences learned from creating and designing collaboratives as an environment for both creativity and leadership to emerge. The intent is to offer guidance on how to design successful collaboratives with leadership engines that produce rapid and sustained transformational results.

Leadership is easy to notice if you're looking for it.

To illustrate the importance of leadership, we'll provide two experiences from everyday life. In one, a leadership dynamic was present and in the other it was absent. The distinction was real, observable and impacted results.

A customer took shirts to be cleaned at a neighborhood laundry. One of the shirts had an ink stain. The customer asked the owner if special attention could be given to removing the stain. The owner said, "Yes, we can do that." She put tape on the stain, put the marked stained shirt in the bag with the other shirts, and wrote a note on the ticket. The customer left with a commitment and confidence that some effort would be made. The owner was in action with system and method.

Weeks later, the same customer was back with more shirts and a new stain. Behind the counter was a clerk. The customer asked if special attention could be given to removing the new stain. The clerk said, "I don't know," put all the shirts in the bag and handed the customer the ticket with no notation. The customer didn't get a commitment. The responder was doing transactions and just a job, not looking for possibilities and opportunities.

The necessary action to remove the ink stain wasn't about better practices, case controls, randomization or better research study design—it was about a leadership choice to act on the customer's need for having the stain treated and removed. "Best practices" to achieve this particular desired result have been known for decades. The key element here is not education—it's leadership commitment and visible actions to achieve the goal.

This is a day-to-day example of how behavior, including improvement projects, can be viewed through a leadership lens. This isn't a "research lens." The purpose of using a leadership lens in a collaborative is to create less rote behavior and more leadership behavior. A successful collaborative means creating a vibrant, engaging and meaningful space for participants to generate and be recognized for their natural leadership, talents, actions and achievements. Collaborative architects and leaders need to be looking for and surfacing this leadership and action.

"The true task of leadership is not to put greatness in to humanity,
but to elicit it, since the greatness is already there."
—John Buchan

In the Moment Leadership Spurs Improvements in National Organ Donation Referrals

The behaviors we want often show up in spontaneous and unexpected ways. In an Organ Donation collaborative one of the key strategies in the change package was called "early referral and rapid response." This means the hospital calls the Organ Procurement Organization (OPO) early in the process of identifying a patient as a potential donor. The intent is to bring the coordinator into work with the family as early as possible. The more time the coordinator has with the family, the greater the trust and the more likely the donation. This dynamic was very clear and was proven to be effective (Shafer, et al., 2008)[1].

Early in the collaborative a panel was discussing the need to adopt "early referral and rapid response" and calling for teams to adopt it. An intensive care unit (ICU) doctor stood to comment: "As a doctor I understand the policy being recommended, but I disagree. I cannot ethically comply. I cannot decide that the patient I am trying to save is close to imminent death. I cannot stop seeking recovery, and then call the OPO acknowledging that there is no hope." The response was heartfelt and emotional. Many in the room applauded.

The staff could sense that many participants in the room were on the verge of moving away from a very powerful practice. Rejection could deter the pathway toward the goal of increasing national organ donation rates from 50 percent to 75 percent[2]. This was a defining moment and a teaching moment. A positive voice was needed.

Suddenly another participant member of a hospital/OPO team stood and addressed the large crowd: "We have encountered this position with doctors in some hospitals. They feel very strongly about it. We worked with them to keep their focus on the patient recovery, while at the same time enabling 'early referral and rapid response' to happen." Suddenly the energy in the room shifted as the new speaker generated possibilities and opportunities: "Our solution was to create a set of objective 'clinical triggers' that would automatically generate hospital outreach to the OPO—things like whether there had been discussions with the patient's family about discontinuing life support, the results of brain flow tests and other objective indicators."

Other collaborative teams immediately asked if their clinical triggers could be shared. The answer was, "Of course, yes." At Learning Session 1 on Sept. 12, 2003 in Washington, D.C., nearly 100 collaborative teams from OPOs and the nation's largest trauma centers made a leadership choice to share, test and adapt the systematic collaborative-wide use of clinical triggers to support the "early referral, rapid response" change package strategy.

The answer was in the room. The leadership style of the event enabled issues to surface and encouraged creative response with the aim in mind, to increase life-saving organ donation rates. Embracing the concern, hearing solutions from the floor, valuing the concerns and the solutions, and acting on them in real time helped to set the stage for the vibrant, inclusive spirit and "all teach all learn" way of being that became a defining condition of this initiative. A leadership act in the right moment created forward momentum.

It's important to examine national collaboratives in healthcare through the leadership lens. Based on more than a decade of experience leading large national quality improvement initiatives, the authors believe that this is the single most important element in effective collaborative design. The question, "What can you do to catalyze more concerted leadership and clinical actions?" increases the odds that leaders emerge and leadership speech and actions will happen.

Leadership behavior of participants is key to the success of a collaborative. The leadership is there; collaboratives have to create the conditions that empower it.

The logic is simple. If you want large-scale system transformation you have to involve lots of people. The more genuine the involvement, the more likely it is that leaders will emerge at any point in time. People want to step forward and will be energized by the possibilities and opportunities generated by bold aims. Commitments, the currency of collaboratives, lead to actions that cause the world to change. Traditional barriers dissolve. Showcasing and celebrating examples of successful actions and behaviors helps to develop leaders worth emulating. Leadership is sparked by the sense of urgency created by tangible stories of patients and caregivers whose lives were profoundly impacted by positive practice reforms. Successful collaboratives are meaningful, intense, fast-paced, content-rich and emotional.

There are six elements of effective large-scale collaborative design:

1. Play big.
2. See and compare change as it happens.
3. Count and convey commitments.
4. Achieve all-in action.
5. Acknowledge people.
6. Make it urgent.

Each of these elements is integral to the design of a blueprint for a successful collaborative. Each of these elements also involves attributes of leadership.

1. Play Big.

Create genuine involvement across every sector and encourage participation to produce a critical mass of engaged leaders. Large-scale collaboratives spread best practices rapidly across many organizations. The entire collaborative must move in the same positive direction. Create a climate that promotes involvement at every level.

Here's an example: The Partnership for Patients (PfP) campaign's aims of reducing preventable hospital acquired conditions by 40 percent and 30-day readmissions by 20 percent were established at a major press event in the National Press Club (HHS) in April 2011. Former HHS Secretary Kathleen Sebelius; former CMS Administrator Don Berwick, M.D.; and leaders from the American Hospital Association, the National Business Group on Health, Honeywell Corporation, the National Partnership for Women and Families, Blue Cross Blue Shield, and other public and private organizations joined the HHS Secretary and the CMS Administrator in committing to these compelling aims.

Over the initial three-year period, numerous HHS and other government agencies participated in weekly meetings to develop alignment and commitments to support the campaign's bold aims. Similarly, CMS and the National Quality Forum (NQF) convened regularly with more than 40 national associations, payers, patient and consumer organizations to generate and track commitments, actions and progress. The American College of Surgeons (ACS), the American Nurses Association (ANA), the Institute for Patient and Family Centered Care (IPFCC), the Joint Commission (JC), Johnson & Johnson and many others became active stakeholders. The nation's hospital safety system was engaged.

This inclusive approach was successful. "Together, HENs recruited over 70 percent of U.S. short stay acute care hospitals (over 3,700 hospitals) to participate with them in the campaign, which account for about 80 percent of U.S. acute care admissions. A second round of hospital recruitment, underway in early 2014 by HENs, promises to further increase the scale of the campaign."[3] An integral feature of powerful aims like those above is that they create systems. Traditional thinking runs in the other direction—that you have to "get ready" and build systems first so that you can pursue aims.

People and organizations attracted to the aims voluntarily commit to them, and then begin to self-align their resources, people, programs and platforms to support the aims. These types of actions create systems. President Kennedy declared, "First, I believe that this nation should commit itself to achieving the goal, before this decade is out, of landing a man on the moon and returning him safely to the earth."[4] This powerful aim caused amazing alignment and system-building throughout the government, the scientific community, the fledgling computer industry, as well as other parts of society. It's hard to imagine designing a "trial" to "test" whether establishing this aim "works," using a counterfactual. Some parties will join in the aim, and some will not. But, the aim is either achieved in the time stated, or it is not. In this case, the aim was achieved.

The AHRQ Scorecard is a powerful example of how the PfP aims created systems. The Scorecard was created by HHS as an independent, integrated, scientific way to measure patient safety nationally across 28 different harm areas, focusing especially on nine key harms targeted by the PfP. It was established to create a pre-existing baseline in 2010 and to track national progress in the same way in 2011, 2012, 2013, 2014 and beyond. Defined this way, the aim described a future that would guide all participants in creating the system that would deliver it. The integration of 28 harm areas into one composite and one aim was revolutionary[5].

The national scorecard was not an attributional design (comparing hospitals with intervention to hospitals without intervention) because an entire national system was being transformed and there were multiple interventions in place. Improvements on the 28 harm efforts reflected the work of federal agencies, private partners, states, professional groups, stakeholder organizations and ongoing improvement efforts. It helped coalesce an ensemble of players into forming a new national system. The collaborative aim and its scorecard were an umbrella for a grand synthesis of many improvement efforts that would result in safe hospitals everywhere and always. This new national measurement system (i.e., annual audit of 30,000 medical records sampled from selected U.S. hospitals) established a baseline of 145 harms per 1,000 discharges in 2010, and has used the same methodology to track hospital harm every year since 2010. The AHRQ Scorecard process has documented a reduction to 121 harms per 1,000 patient discharges in 2013—an overall reduction of 17 percent, and a 39 percent reduction in preventable harm[6].

2. See and Compare Change as It Happens.

Create a compelling vision and contrast it with reality. This will trigger leaders to generate possibilities, opportunities and commitments.

Collaboratives create positive change that can be seen and experienced together in real time. The bold aim prepares us to watch for significant improvements. Aiming in order to generate change sounds like this: Did you know that out of every 1,000 patients admitted to a hospital, 145 will experience an avoidable harm? That's a lot of harming. Watch those harms because we're going to reduce preventable harms by 40 percent over the next three years.

Collaboratives work by helping participants see and experience desired change as it happens and then apply the best practices that they've observed. Counting, measuring and reporting the metrics of incremental changes should be acknowledged and rewarded. Rapid cycle improvement depends upon effective measurement and evaluation to demonstrate timely (i.e., weekly and monthly) changes in performance (using run charts).

Utilizing real-time tracking provides the ability to identify high performers and evaluate their breakthrough improvement factors. Likewise, collaboratives can identify negative outliers and provide timely support and guidance. The collaborative's motto should be "chase the high performers and leave no one behind." These conversations, with the high and low performers, help to identify opportunities and disseminate best practice in a rapid manner.

The following story is about what it looks like to help generate, surface and spread high performance.

Reducing Catheter Associated Urinary Tract Infections

In the PfP, more than 3,700 hospitals were working on a full agenda of patient safety threats, one of which was catheter-associated urinary tract infections (CAUTI). National data revealed increasing rates for CAUTI. There are multiple risk factors for infections for hospitalized patients with urinary catheters. The risk of CAUTI increases the longer the catheter is in place. In many cases, the use and duration of catheter placement is linked to nursing and patient convenience[7,8]. CAUTIs are painful and unnecessary, but deterring unnecessary catheter use has been an ongoing widespread challenge.

The Dignity Health Hospital Engagement Network (HEN) made a leadership-level decision that their 36 acute care hospitals would significantly reduce CAUTI rates as part of their participation in the national PfP campaign. Infection preventionists and nursing leaders used a three-step approach:

1. Stop the unnecessary use of catheters.
2. If one is used, remove it as soon as possible.
3. If it stays in, document the reason why in the chart.

Dignity implemented the policy with system and method across the entire network of hospitals, involving hundreds of daily actions by nurses and other clinicians resulting in significant, systemwide decreases (Figure 1).

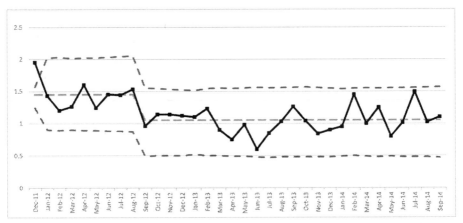

Source: Dignity Health HEN Monthly Report, November, 2014

Figure 1. Dignity Health Catheter Associated Urinary Tract Infections (CAUTI) per 1,000 Catheter Days (Hospital-Wide)

Dignity's accomplishment was featured on the collaborative's national stage, giving Dignity's team the opportunity to help 3,700 hospitals take actions to improve. Frontline leadership by infection preventionists, nurses and others was acknowledged, parsed for effective practices, and rapidly deployed.

3. Count Commitments.

Convene participants in high-energy events, and generate commitments through teachable and replicable leadership style.

Collaboratives move forward through frequent learning events ("pacing events") where participants convene for what Institute for Healthcare Improvement (IHI) refers to as "all teach, all learn." The intent is three-fold:

1. Experience the overall progress of the collaborative.
2. Share tangible team progress and successful practices.
3. Commit to take informed, specific, additional rapid actions toward the aims. Each learning event is followed by an action period.

To highlight the need to design events that generate commitments, we refer to the learning sessions as "pacing events." They set the pace of teams toward the aim. Pacing events can be a valuable way to motivate or reset a campaign.

Participants use speech acts (declarations, assertions, effective questions, requests and offers) to build relationships and generate action steps. Throughout the event, teams stand and commit to specific actions they'll apply in the next time period to advance toward the aim(s). This public declaration is a powerful process of learning, inspiration and accountability. Teams leave confident in their plans as part of a larger community committed to learning and improvement, moving together toward a common countable vision of the future. Participants are expected to engage and participate in the pacing events throughout the collaborative. Leadership of these events should intentionally focus on using them as engines for generating commitments to action. If you leave an event without commitments, then the leadership is not effective.

On March 1-2, 2012, early in the PfP campaign, leaders of the 26 newly designated Hospital Engagement Networks (HENs) met with each other and the CMS team. The intent was to identify next steps on the shared aims in a way that would propel teams forward. As leaders convened, the sense in the air was one of excitement, eagerness and seeking to connect—all tempered with a growing realization that this newly formed community of practice had two huge accountabilities, including: achieving a 40 percent reduction across nine patient preventable harm areas in U.S. hospitals by the end of calendar year 2014. This is a BIG aim[9].

CMS staff presented three key requests to the HENs:

1. Implement sprints in each network to generate a HEN-wide "First Focus" result by August 2012—reportable real results in six months!
2. Implement a campaign-wide sprint in all networks together to substantially reduce early elective deliveries by August 2012—not one of the original nine harms, so this broadened an already BIG aim!

3. Commit to hitting a series of shared management milestones over the next several months—accelerate the rate at which hospitals are moving forward!

The first two requests were informed by clear guidance from the HHS secretary, CMS administrator, and CMS Innovation Center director. For example, based on clear evidence that early elective deliveries (EED) prior to 39 weeks gestation are quite harmful to infants, coupled with further estimates that the national EED rate was 9 percent, the secretary and her team set a national goal of reducing EEDs to less than 5 percent. CMS Administrator Marilyn Tavenner called on the HENs to generate EED HEN-wide results in the first six months by August 2012. The American College of Obstetrics and Gynecology and the March of Dimes (two PfP partners) joined with HHS in committing to the goal.

The tone of the meeting quickly became even more serious as HENs absorbed the goals and related requests. More work? Faster progress?

After the initial request, questions, and many expressed concerns, the teams went to work using three powerful "Effective Questions," including: What excites me about these requests? What are the good things about adding EED work to our shared portfolio? What offers can I make to this collaborative network to advance on this aim?

After 15 minutes for processing, the room returned with answers, including:

- The practice for reducing EED rates in hospitals is proven, effective and crystal clear: Establish a "hard stop" policy to prevent scheduling of any EEDs in the hospital.
- Adding to the aim is a good thing, a sign of the secretary's confidence in and support for the HEN network.
- Taking on EEDs is an opportunity to say "yes" to the leading government health

71

officials, gain quick wins, and show the strength of the new HEN network.

- Adding EEDs to the network's aim is a good thing because this is the pattern we want for the long term – turning to this network to help move the nation to quick results on beneficial quality improvement actions.

- Most important of all, reducing EEDs is better for babies!

Further, some leaders affirmed that the 5 percent EED goal was achievable and could happen quickly. Ann Hendrich, the vice president for Quality and Safety at Ascension Health, affirmed that their network of 70+ hospitals (who cared for diverse and underserved populations) had already achieved a low EED rate of approximately 3 percent (2012).

Maulik Joshi, associate executive vice president at the American Hospital Association (AHA) and president of the Health Research & Educational Trust (HRET), the research and education affiliate of the AHA and leader of the largest HEN, noted that the AHA Board was considering commitment to a policy recommendation for EED hard stops in all hospitals (which later occurred). Several other HENs then stepped up publicly and offered to add the EED work to already planned work on obstetrical harm.

The tide had shifted. Leaders were stepping up to the request in real time. To firm up the emerging plans, each HEN leader and team members publicly declared their EED goal and planned next steps and then signed a commitment chart that was produced in real time. It was incredibly energizing, substantive and authentic. Teams left in action with clear targets and a plan for executing them rapidly.

So what happened? By December 2014, 1,943 birthing hospitals had reduced their EED rate from 10 percent to 3 percent, resulting in an estimated 34,446 fewer babies potentially harmed by EEDs. National data showed an even greater reduction of 118,113 EEDs averted (Figure 2).

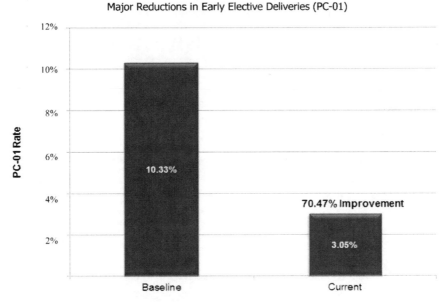

Source: HEN-reported data submitted November 2014

Figure 2. Collaborative achieved big reductions in EEDs

Leadership can be spontaneous or developed as a result of learning and reflection. Some HENs didn't initially declare an EED goal. Even though they were already a national leader, the Ascension HEN later reported that they were declaring a new systemwide goal of zero(!) EEDs. Within a year, the Ascension EED rate dropped below 1 percent. This is national leadership where the best-in-class challenged themselves to attain even higher levels of performance. Initially, a commitment to new, unprecedented levels of safety didn't seem realistic to them. Upon reflection, they committed to and achieved the goal (Figure 3).

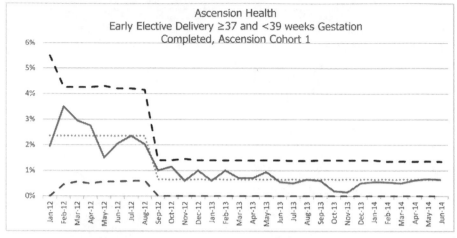

Figure 3. Ascension Health System: Early Elective Deliveries

The work done at the two-day event shows the power of using events to generate requests, offers, commitments, actions and results. This includes the power to "break through" to even higher levels of performance, previously not thought possible.

4. Achieve All-in Action.

Introduce simple generative action methods, and use them to overcome the barriers to leadership action. Teams on the ground are expected to move forward relentlessly and show short-term progress and results. How do these behaviors happen in a volunteer environment when the teams are made up of clinicians who are already busy, many of them with a significant patient case load and little improvement experience?

People rarely say "no" to a request for action. Instead, they avoid saying "yes" by referring to the triangle of resistance. It sounds like this:

"I'm too busy."
"I don't have permission."
"I have to get ready first."

Time, permission and readiness seem reasonable at first glance, and out of the control of the responder. These may look like organization-imposed constraints, but they're not.

Collaboratives can do many things to effectively disarm these responses. For example: Have each organization's executives sign a letter committing to the collaborative and its aims. Even then, the resistance triangle may remain a challenge due to inherent personal reactions and learned behaviors. Collaborative leadership must diagnose and manage (respond to) the symptoms of participant fear and lethargy when they occur. Collaboratives can be designed to break the triangle and make action easier to launch.

Such techniques enable teams to start and build momentum. We recently encountered a powerful example of this in an innovative collaborative funded by CMS called Leading Edge Advanced Practice Topics (LEAPT). Where, in addition to working on the 10 patient safety areas of focus, six HENs are pursuing Leading Edge Advance Practice Topics (LEAPT) that will enhance overall progress on the Partnership for Patients' goals.

CMS conducted a competitive process to select six HENs participating under PfP to address a set of serious but underdeveloped safety topics. Each HEN received funding to enable an intense effort to address a subset of 11 advanced topics that included: Severe Sepsis and Septic Shock, Clostridium Difficile, Worker Safety and others. At the onset of LEAPT the HENs had a traditional linear mindset. They were laying out a traditional sequence of steps to address the topics individually, or one at a time. CMS staff made a request to do what at first sounded impractical and maybe impossible: produce compelling improvement results in pilot hospital safety immediately and demonstrate rapid spread across HENs within months. This wasn't a grant condition or contract negotiation; it was a leadership request.

These "advanced topics" in avoidable harms were so-called because there wasn't a well-developed body of knowledge on how to prevent them. They didn't have the historical measurement systems that the original 10 PfP topics had. It felt like there needed to be more research, testing, development, prototypes, publishing, peer review, and then of course, dissemination and adoption. There were a lot of comments regarding "getting ready," "we don't have enough time," and "do we have permission?" At the same time, the HENs were drawn to the urgency of these topics and the request. They saw possibilities in the improvement concept of rapid cycle development. On every topic it turned out that there was an experience base to draw on and willing hospitals ready to take on the safety topic. In only 15 months, the six HENs identified, developed and adapted interventions, set aims, measured progress, achieved initial results, and initiated spread across the larger network of 3,700 hospitals. These remarkable achievements occurred because the HENs made a leadership choice to implement around a proven rapid-cycle methodology. They made this choice even though the network didn't seem "ready."

5. Acknowledge Leaders.

Model and celebrate positive leadership, action and behaviors, and bring forward successful people to share their leadership concepts for change. Collaboratives help to identify and spread best evidence-based practice principles. They're most effective when the collaborative implements a systemwide culture that promotes commitment, measurement, transparent reporting, learning and action.

Often, knowledge is thought of as published articles, toolkits, operating manuals, applications, a software program or a written body of information. This isn't the case with a collaborative. Collaboratives move too fast and with unique conditions for local implementation; it's more "adapt" than "adopt." It's more "just in time" learning than "turnkey" installation and instruction. For collaboratives, knowledge is best gathered, analyzed and deployed through frontline faculty leaders who are experienced and engaged in the practice settings.

Start with a "change package "containing "ideas" that teams can test. The content comes from the scientific literature and, especially, the real-world experiences and improvements of innovative and successful front-line practitioners—practitioners who have the data to document their success[10]. HRSA used the change-package approach for the Patient Safety and Clinical Pharmacy Services Collaborative to reduce ADEs and potential ADEs in primary care[11,12,13]. Teams visited multiple high-performing, cutting-edge sites identified from the literature and analyses of performance data. The site visit teams used the local examples to produce a working draft of the change package, and identified candidates to play leadership roles as faculty and coaches. Collaboratives are truly successful when all teams bring forth leadership voices that are committed to successful transformation of practice.

6. Make it Urgent.

Link it to life. Leadership is emboldened and empowered when the desired end is linked to the reality that healthcare impacts lives. Engage patients and families to increase the relevance, learning and emotion that leads to urgency and action.

Collaboratives are often voluntary efforts. Organizations join collaboratives because they believe the topic is important. There's always some initial level of commitment to the desired transformation. Health is relevant and important to us all.

But thinking something is important isn't the same as thinking the change is urgent or even achievable. As leaders and participants in these voluntary, important initiatives, how do we generate and sustain the energy and commitment necessary to really make them work?

It's imperative to maintain a collective focus on patients and families. Sharing actual patient cases puts a face and a heart on the issue. Applying this perspective helps to instill a sense of urgency in the pursuit for change and improvement. Integrating patients and families into the work of collaboratives can make a dramatic difference. They become critical voices and partners in the work by contributing an essential "reality check" to the process. This function was driven home early in the work of the HHS PfP collaborative. Although more than 3,700 hospitals were engaged into the partnership, many participating hospitals would only commit to working on a few of the nine harm areas. They were saying they had to be realistic and set priorities.

The collaborative wasn't designed to improve several harms, but rather to transform hospitals to become safe systems of care. All harms must be addressed. It would be easy to launch a few one-off projects and leave the underlying system in place. The PfP leaders insisted that working on all the harms was necessary to help teams force changes in their organizational culture and systems. Hospital teams, confronted with the challenging difficulties of "system change," were pushing back.

Patients and families organizations and advocates were partners in the PfP. They saw this tension and conceptual argument, and grounded their strong feedback and leadership direction in much more practical, human terms. In a key national webinar attended by thousands of caregivers, an outspoken patient put it quite plainly: "What patient wants to go to a hospital that's good at preventing one or two forms of harm?" The polite but serious debate over setting priorities that had been ongoing, stopped. It didn't start again. Patients made the aim come alive as a moral imperative. A campaign ethos became established.

In retrospect, patients told HHS the initiative should have been named the Partnership with Patients (PwP).

Patient Leadership Saves Lives

Consider the example of Susan McVey Dillon. Hundreds of physicians, nurses and organ-donation coordinators met Sue at a collaborative learning session in Dallas in January 2004. Sue told the audience about the tragic climbing accident of her teenage son, Michael, who suffered a devastating brain injury from which he would never recover. After several days of intensive medical attention and steadily worsening medical tests, Sue and her family learned that Michael would never walk, never speak again, couldn't breathe on his own, and would never regain consciousness. They made the heart-wrenching decision to remove life support.

In a moment of compassion for other mothers, Sue inquired about the possibility that her son could become a life-saving organ donor. She wanted other moms to experience what she could not—the chance to bring their loved one home from the hospital. Sue learned that the hospital caring for her son didn't have a policy to permit the procedure called "donation after cardiac death" (DCD donation). They insisted that the hospital "figure it out." To the credit of the enlightened and competent hospital staff and team at the organ procurement organization in Philadelphia, they did just that. They figured it out and Michael became a life-saving organ donor. Several years later, Sue and her family even met "Santos," the young father of two children from Puerto Rico, whose life was saved by Michael's gift of life.

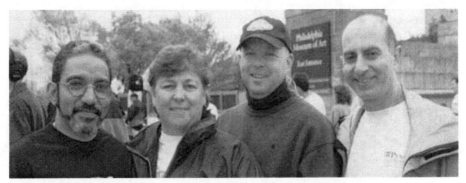

Left to right are Santos, Susan McVey Dillon, John Edwards of Gift of Life, and Transplant Surgeon Avi Shaked, M.D.

Sue looked out over the audience that day in January 2004 and reported that most of the nearly 100 large trauma centers represented in the room didn't have policies in place to enable donation after cardiac death. She said, "I'm a teacher of young special needs children. In my classroom, the words 'I can't' and 'I won't' aren't permitted. When it comes to enabling donation after cardiac death in your hospitals, I expect no less from you."

The impact of this family member was profound. The caregivers in that room, their hospitals and the nation's entire organ donation system responded. According the official Scientific Registry of Transplant Recipients publicly posted annual report, over the course of 2004 and subsequent years, DCD donation in the United States more than doubled, increasing from 214 in 2003 to 538 in 2006.[14] Many hundreds of lives were saved or enhanced as a result of the DCD increases that Sue and the participants of the collaborative helped to generate.

To create the essential urgency and impact of your collaborative, there's one design principle to keep at the forefront: Engage patients and families.

Conclusion

Well-designed collaboratives work. Large, national collaboratives like the PfP, the Organ Donation Breakthrough Collaborative, the Advancing Excellence Campaign, the Patient Safety and Clinical Pharmacy Services Collaborative, and others have made immense contributions to life-saving and life-enhancing results (Figure 4).

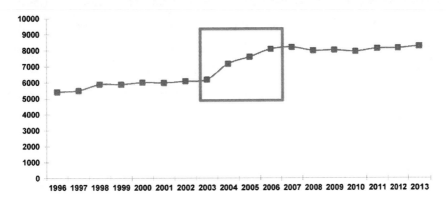

Major National Increases in Number Of Organ Donors Per Year: 2002 to 2006

Figure 4. This run chart shows the tremendous impact of the Organ Donation Breakthrough Collaborative.

Similarly, there have been tremendous national reductions in patient harm from 2010 through 2013. Based on the Agency for Healthcare Research on Quality (AHRQ) National Scorecard, the Department of Health and Human Services estimated that 50,000 fewer patients died in hospitals and approximately $12 billion in healthcare costs were saved as a result of a reduction in hospital-acquired conditions from 2010 to 2013[15].

This progress toward a safer healthcare system occurred during a period of concerted attention by hospitals throughout the country to reduce adverse events. The efforts were due in part to provisions of the Affordable Care Act, such as Medicare payment incentives to improve the quality of care and the HHS PfP initiative.

Highly coordinated and centralized alignment is very likely to have been a major contributor to these results. Preliminary estimates show that in total, hospital patients experienced 1.3 million fewer hospital-acquired conditions from 2010 to 2013. This translates to a 17 percent decline in hospital-acquired conditions over the three-year period and a 39 percent reduction in preventable harm.

Detailed information on how these results were calculated are available at: http://www.ahrq.gov/professionals/quality-patient-safety/pfp/interimhacrate2013.html

We have much more to learn about the leadership, behaviors, actions and mechanisms through which these types of outcome results can be produced. Over the years, the "research lens" has assisted us greatly in identifying the best interventions to use, supported by the evidence.

To reach the next level of achievement in safety and quality, it's very likely we'll need to learn more about how to expertly blend the "research lens" with what we've described here: the "leadership lens." What we do know is that when hundreds or thousands of organizations with committed caregivers come together and genuinely commit to bold, measureable aims and go into concerted action together—supported by patients and the other ingredients of a well-designed collaborative improvement effort—outcomes that were once thought "impossible" become possible.

This chapter was prepared or accomplished by Dr. Paul McGann, Dennis Wagner, Dr. Daniel Buffington, and Dr. John Scanlon in their personal capacity. The opinions expressed in this publication are the author's own and do not reflect the view of the Centers for Medicare & Medicaid Services, the Department of Health and Human Services, or the United States government.

[1] Shafer, T., Wagner, D., Chessare, J., Schall, M., McBride, V., Zampiello, F., et al. (2008). US Organ Donation Breakthrough Collaborative Increases Organ Donation. *Crit Care Nurs Q , 31* (3), 190-210. 194.

[2] Shafer, T. et al. pg. 191.

[3] Clarkwest, A., Chen, A., Higgins, M., Cheh, V., Zurovac, J., Kranker, K., et al. (2014, 07 10). Project Evaluation Activity in Support of Partnership for Patients: Task 2 Evaluation Progress Report. *PfP PEC: Evaluation Profress Report ,* 1-71.

[4] Kennedy, J. F. (2004, 5 4). NASA - Excerpt from the 'Special Message to the Congress on Urgent National Needs'. *Speech to Congress, 5/25/61.* NASA.

[5] Hackbarth, A., Munier, W., Jordan, J., Richards, C., Brennan, N., Wagner, D., et al. (2014). An Overview of Measurement Activities in the Partnership for Patients. *J Patient Saf: PfP , 0* (0), 1-8. 2.

[6] Efforts To Improve Patient Safety Result in 1.3 Million Fewer Patient Harms. (2014, December). *Agency for Healthcare Research and Quality.*

[7] Hazzard, Blass, Ettinger, Halter, & Ouslander. (1998). Chapter 62. In *Principles of Geriatric Medicine and Gerontology* (4th edition ed., pp. 832-833). TX: McGraw-Hill.

[8] Kane, R., Ouslander, J., Abrass, I., & Resnick, B. (1994). Chapter 6: Incontinence. In *Essentials of Clinical Geriatrics, 3rd edition* (3rd Edition ed., pp. 187-189). McGraw-Hill Education.

[9] Hackbarth, et al. pg 1.

[10] Improvement, I. f. (2004). The Breakthrough Series IHI's Collaborative Model for Achieving Breakthrough Improvement. *White Papers: Innovation Series , 3-17.*

[11] *US Department of Health and Human Services: HSRA.* Retrieved from Patient Safety and Clinical Pharmacy Services Collaborative (PSPC): Communities of Practice: http://www.hrsa.gov/communitiesofpractice/AtaGlance/patientsafety.pdf.

[12] Pedley, K. (n.d.). HRSA's Patient Safety and Clinical Pharmacy Services Collaborative (PSPC). *US Department of Health and Human Services: HRSA.* http://www.hrsa.gov/ruralhealth/media/508ehrincentive052609.pdf

[13] Management, A. f. (2012). *The PSPC 2012 National Performance Story.* Retrieved from The Patient Safety and Clinical Pharmacy Services Collaborative: http://medsmatter.org/the-patient-safety-and-clinical-pharmacy-services-collaborative-2012-national-performance-story/

[14] US Department of Health and Human Services. (2006). *2006 Annual Report.* Retrieved from Welcome to the 2006 OPTN / SRTR Annual Report: Transplant Data 1996-2005: http://www.srtr.org/annual_reports/archives/2006/2006_Annual_Report/default.htm

[15] Efforts to Improve Patient Safety, 2014.

CHAPTER 5

Collaborative Governance–
Three Case Studies

By Lucy A. Savitz, Ph.D., MBA, Sam R. Watson, MSA, CPPS
and Diane Stewart, MBA

Introduction

When engaging multiple organizations and stakeholders in collaboratives, it's
important to give early consideration to how the effort will be governed. This chapter
will address governance through the experiences of three large-scale collaboratives.

The chapter will explore the three different approaches to governance
through case studies for the High Value Healthcare Collaborative, the Michigan
Health and Hospital Association and the California Quality Collaborative.
Each case study will explore four questions:

1. What's the impetus for collaboration? This question helps identify who
   should be engaged to provide direction and oversight to a collaborative.
2. How do you determine the structure, formal or informal, and will it
   evolve over time? Collaboratives are organic, in the sense that as the
   stakeholders learn and test approaches, the complexity changes. It's also
   important to consider the structure from the standpoint of data sharing.
   Determining the mechanism for how data will be collected, protected
   and shared is a fundamental element.

3. How does governance provide the means to prioritize and evaluate the collaborative and the projects or interventions deployed? The potential for scope creep is a constant threat to any project; having a governance structure that determines scope and resources is important to maintain focus.

4. How should collaboratives be funded? While this issue will be addressed in greater detail elsewhere in this book, the three examples provided in this chapter will give the reader a perspective about the need for diversity in sustainability.

Case Study: High Value Healthcare Collaborative

By Lucy A. Savitz, Ph.D., MBA

"None of us is as smart as all of us."

—Warren Bennis and Patricia Ward Biederman, "Genius: The Secrets of Creative Collaboration, page 1"

High Value Healthcare Collaborative (HVHC) is a voluntary, member-led organization based on trusted, working relationships among healthcare delivery system leaders. Representing a cross-section of the healthcare industry (i.e., geography, teaching status, size, religious affiliation and payers, including both critical access and safety net hospitals), it was formed to adapt to a complex, changing environment.

Dr. Jack Wennberg and others from the Dartmouth Institute had informally brought together leaders from Mayo Clinic and Intermountain Healthcare who were identified by the Dartmouth Atlas as low-cost, high-quality providers. In the fall of

2009, with Washington policymakers focused on healthcare reform, they decided to expand and formalize a group to establish a collective voice for delivery systems interested in leading the way on healthcare transformation and payment reform.

Creating a collective voice and safe environment for shared learning wasn't a new idea. Organizational scientists have talked about the promising notion of strategic alliances as a vehicle for health services innovation[1]. As member organizations executed a memoranda of understanding, the press dubbed HVHC the "dream team."[2]

Beginning with five founding members—peaking at one point at 19—HVHC currently has 14 delivery system members (see sidebar). This fluctuation in membership is consistent with a living systems theory of organizational behavior whereby the collaborative can be thought of as a living social organism—not static—that expands and contracts based on the changing needs and priorities of the group and its members over its lifespan.[3]

HVHC founding members were committed to using a data-driven approach in shared learning. They decided to use a centralized model for data sharing, creating a data trust that was and continues to be managed by the HVHC Program Management Office. Issues around data privacy, access and transparency, together with policies and procedures for governance, led to hiring independent counsel to execute a master collaborative agreement (MCA). More details on the MCA[4], the data submission process[5], and an example of comparative work[6] have been published elsewhere.

HVHC Membership, 8/1/15

- Baylor Scott & White
- Beth Israel Deaconess Medical Center
- Dartmouth Hitchcock
- Denver Health
- Eastern Maine Health System
- Hawaii Pacific Health
- Intermountain Healthcare
- Mayo Clinic
- North Shore-LIJ Health System
- Providence Health & Services
- Sinai Health System
- University of California, San Diego
- University of Iowa
- Virginia Mason Medical Center

Great groups have to invent a leadership style and structure that suits them[7]. The founding members of HVHC constituted a steering committee, holding decision-making authority for the collaborative, that informed senior leaders from newly added member organizations who served on the executive committee. HVHC is currently evolving its governance structure as a member-led organization that's more inclusive in representation of all member organizations in response to recommendations from a recent task force review. The steering committee remains in place as authorized in the MCA.

A non-traditional board structure includes five committees—Finance, Discovery and Dissemination, Data Governance, Scientific and Advocacy—and an overarching chair. Aside from Finance, each committee includes an elected chair and vice chair who are required to be members of the executive committee to be board eligible. Each of these committees has focused program areas supporting collaborative work that are led by staff from member organizations. Board committees and programs are supported by staff from the Program Management Office based at the Dartmouth Institute; and the CEO of the Program Management Office reports to the chair of the board.

Core funding for HVHC comes from membership dues; supplemental funding for planned activities comes from Centers for Medicare and Medicaid Innovation and the Laura and John Arnold Foundation via two in-progress awards. The closely related AHRQ ACTION is a subset of HVHC member organizations poised to conduct rapid cycle research, using HVHC as a dissemination vehicle for evidence-based, best practice discoveries.

As a member-led organization, HVHC aligns with the strategic priorities of member delivery systems. Other factors contributing to its success are leveraging pre-existing relationships, starting small then expanding, creating a safe environment for data-driven shared learning, establishing and evolving a governance structure that meets HVHC's changing needs, and being responsive by demonstrating value to members.

Case Study: Michigan Health & Hospital Association (MHA)

By Sam R. Watson, MSA, CPPS

In 2003, the Michigan Health & Hospital Association (MHA) Board of Trustees directed the association to aid members in the improvement of quality and patient safety. The direction was given based in part on the Institute of Medicine's report on patient safety, "To Err is Human,"[8] and "Crossing the Quality Chasm"[9] report on healthcare quality, as well as poor ranking in various quality metrics. As a result, the MHA Keystone Center patient safety organization was created as a division of MHA Health Foundation.

Shortly after the launch of the MHA Keystone Center, the Agency for Healthcare Research and Quality (AHRQ) announced funding opportunities for patient safety initiatives, an opportunity that gave life to the newly formed center, with more than 70 hospitals ultimately participating in the Keystone Intensive Care Unit (ICU) collaborative.

Since the initial ICU collaborative, MHA Keystone Center's work has blossomed to include improvement efforts in labor and delivery, emergency, surgery, sepsis and care transitions. In addition, the MHA Keystone Center became a federally certified patient safety organization and works under contract with the Centers for Medicare and Medicaid Services as a Hospital Engagement Network (HEN). In all cases, the original call to action by the MHA Board of Trustees to lead Michigan hospitals to the highest levels of care has held as the North Star or point of focus.

While the MHA Keystone Center, working with Dr. Peter Pronovost and his team at Johns Hopkins Hospital, managed the day-to-day operations of the ICU collaborative, it formed an advisory team to garner input and guidance from ICU physicians and nurses to better implement evidence-based interventions in daily work routines and patient care.

This advisory group was sufficient for the Keystone ICU collaborative, but as the number of collaboratives grew, an advisory board was needed to provide a broader strategic perspective. Because the MHA Keystone Center initially operated under the MHA Health Foundation, the Keystone advisory board didn't have fiduciary responsibilities but rather provided strategic vision and counseled Keystone Center staff on the direction of existing collaboratives as well as consideration of new initiatives.

Keystone purposefully designed the advisory board to be comprised of participants who represent physicians, hospitals and purchasers of care. This diverse board helps the MHA Keystone Center to have a broader perspective when deploying patient safety and quality initiatives.

While the MHA Keystone Center was actively seeking to improve care, President George W. Bush signed the Quality Improvement and Patient Safety Act of 2005 into law. This law called for the creation of patient safety organizations (PSO). The MHA created a PSO as a separate 501(c)(3) nonprofit organization. The MHA PSO and the MHA Keystone Center operated in tandem but distinct from one another for a few years, until both organizations were combined to become a federally certified PSO. The MHA Keystone Center became a wholly owned subsidiary to the MHA Health Foundation with a separate board of directors.

This board, as with the former MHA PSO board, is diverse with hospitals, physicians, nurses, consumers, long-term care and purchasers of care providing fiduciary oversight to the MHA Keystone Center.

Under this organizational design, each collaborative still maintains an advisory committee that represents the disciplines involved in the collaborative. In addition, the MHA Keystone Center added a patient and family advisory council to guide the inclusion of patient and family engagement in all quality and patient safety efforts.

The MHA Keystone Center initially identified two interventions, a marked reduction in central line associated bloodstream infection (CLABSI) within a Johns Hopkins Hospital ICU, based on the results of a publication by Dr. Pronovost, et al.[10]

As a result of early and significant success across the state of Michigan in reducing CLABSI and VAP, clinicians began to ask about Keystone working with them to reduce other infections and eventually make other forms of improvement, such as the use of lean methods and the reduction in early elective deliveries. This resulted in the need to develop a process to determine what new collaborative activities the MHA Keystone Center would undertake as well as how it would address implementation.

To determine what interventions Keystone would seek to implement, it applies a set of four tests:

1. Does the intervention address a large enough problem to engage more than a few hospitals?

2. Is the intervention evidence-based or, at the minimum, does it have a consensus in the medical community?

3. Are there processes or outcome measures directly tied to the intervention?

4. Can the intervention be replicated and spread across a large number of diverse hospitals?

Based on how a given intervention fairs against these tests, the organization proposes to the MHA Keystone board its intent to pilot an intervention or interventions with a small number of facilities to determine its ability to implement and measure in the Michigan setting. A pilot may include three to 10 hospitals representing varied geography or settings (e.g., teaching, non-teaching and rural/urban). Based on the results of the pilot, including feedback from participating hospitals, Keystone would present its intent to enroll more hospitals in a full-fledged collaborative.

The MHA Keystone Center board, as well as its other stakeholders such as funders and participating hospitals, holds the center staff accountable for outcomes. The evaluation of projects has taken many forms, from formal evaluation of ICU and sepsis, to less formal evaluations of improvement demonstrated by a change in pre- and post-measurements.

The first element of evaluation is whether Keystone achieved the aim of the collaborative. For example, in its emergency department (ED) project, Keystone used a lean method to improve patient flow. Metrics captured included door to doctor, left without being seen, left against medical advice, and ED length of stay. These measures were captured and reported to improvement teams as well as the MHA Keystone board and the funder on a routine basis. Medicare discharge data was used in the Keystone ICU project to analyze length of stay and mortality for participating hospitals against a control group[11]. An economic evaluation for the Keystone sepsis project used Medicare charge data to compare septic-shock patient charges of participating hospitals against a control group of non-participants.

The MHA Keystone Center has been funded by an assortment of means over the course of its history. The sources have included federal grants from the Agency for Healthcare Research and Quality, the Centers for Disease Control and Prevention, as well as state government. More recently, the Blue Cross Blue Shield of Michigan, through unrestricted donations and the Centers for Medicare and Medicaid Services have provided significant funding to support to collaborative work in the state. Finally, Michigan hospitals have also supported the work through a subscription.

Since the MHA Keystone Center began, the governance has continued to grow in sophistication. The expansion of the improvement portfolio created a need for strategic oversight and, coupled with the need to be accountable to participants and funders, led to a more formal structure, both organizationally and at a governance level.

Case Study: California Quality Collaborative

By Diane Stewart, MBA

Started in 2007, the California Quality Collaborative (CQC) is a multi-stakeholder healthcare improvement organization whose mission is to advance the quality and efficiency of the outpatient healthcare delivery system in California, generating scalable and measurable improvement in care delivery in ways important to patients, purchasers, providers and health plans. The California Quality Collaborative emerged from a statewide collaborative diabetes improvement project initiated in 2002.

Each year, CQC engages about 1,500 individuals from 200 organizations, mostly medical groups, independent practice associations (IPAs) and clinics, in a variety of programs that range from 90-minute teleconferences to year-long intensive collaboratives to support leadership teams implementing system changes within their organizations to achieve specific measurable goals.

CQC's core funding comes from contributions from the four major health plans—Anthem, Blue Shield, HealthNet and United (Wilson)[12]—sharing a delivery system, outside of Kaiser Permanente, the largest health plan in California, which has a dedicated delivery system. Core funding is augmented by grants from government and private funders.

In 2003, Integrated Healthcare Association (IHA), a leadership group that promotes healthcare quality improvement, accountability and affordability in California, launched the California Pay for Performance program for 225 provider organizations representing 35,000 doctors, based on a publicly reported set of measures for clinical quality, patient experience and health information technology. In the first year, six commercial health plans made performance-based payments based on the common measure set representing care for 6 million patients, making it the largest pay-for-performance (P4P) program in the country.[13]

Immediately, physician groups sought ways to improve their performance on the P4P metrics to earn higher bonus payments from the health plans. The health plans sought ways to compete against Kaiser on the publicly reported P4P measures. The four statewide health plans agreed to contribute funding to CQC based on the reasoning that more improvement is possible by pooling funds to provide one intensive technical assistance program to providers ("strength of signal") than doing it alone. In addition, the statewide provider group organization, California Association of Physician Groups (CAPG), agreed to support the program by promoting its offerings to its membership.

Pacific Business Group on Health (PBGH), a not-for-profit purchaser coalition, historically served as a neutral table for collaborative quality projects in California and led the formation of CQC's multi-stakeholder governance structure. CQC is not incorporated as a separate 501(c)(3) non-profit but is technically a program of PBGH, which administers the funds and hires the staff. The program direction is set by a multi-stakeholder steering committee.

The following are the primary functions of CQC's steering committee[14]:

- Set program priorities, or aims.
- Set funding priorities for programs within the aims and endorse the annual work plan.
- Strengthen the program by linking staff and programs to experts, potential participants and funding sources.
- Require each member of the steering committee to participate in one program, either through a design sub-committee or as a program liaison to the steering committee.

The 21 members of the steering committee are from the following:

- Health plan members (funders)
- Delivery systems (customers)
- Purchasers
- Community agencies
- Partners:
  - Other California-based improvement organizations, including the Quality Innovation Network-Quality Improvement Organization (QIN-QIO)
  - IHA, California's multi-stakeholder measurement and reporting organization
  - CAPG, which represents a large proportion of CQC's customers

To reinforce the collaborative spirit of the program, the two co-chairs of the steering committee always represent a health plan and a provider group. Co-chairs meet at least twice a month with the CQC program director and clinical director (a physician).

The nine-person executive committee meets an additional three times a year to do the following:

- Monitor program performance
- Approve grant applications in excess of $50,000
- Approve members for the steering committee

Governance has not changed significantly over time, except to adjust membership of the steering committee, based on market changes over the years. For instance, as improving transitions of care became increasingly important, CQC added hospital systems to its membership. With Medicaid expansion, CQC adjusted membership to incorporate health plans and providers with Medicaid experience.

Over the years, the steering committee has considered whether to incorporate as a separate 501(c)(3) and so far has decided against it. The current arrangement works in two ways: 1) politically, because PBGH serves as a "neutral table" for competing health plans to discuss improvement priorities with provider groups with whom they often have a contentious relationship, and 2) financially, because PBGH provides the financial security of a larger organization to mitigate the variability in funding levels year to year.

The steering committee's most important function is to set program priorities because there are so many possible improvement initiatives, and statewide improvement requires discipline and focus over years, not just months. Every three years, the steering committee sets the improvement priorities, or aims, for the organization in response to evolving performance-based reimbursement and public reporting initiatives in California and nationally.

Despite health plans being the major funders, the committee sets the aims by a vote of all steering committee members (see sidebar). A recent process included a review of federal and state value-based payment programs across all business lines: Medicare, commercial and Medicaid, including those envisioned by the Affordable Care Act (ACA) in the future. Staff conducts a series of interviews with purchasers, plans and providers to anticipate the most important improvements the market will require of the delivery system in the coming years.

The aims are intended to be the program priorities for three years. At times, the steering committee needs to adjust programming in response to significant changes in performance-based payments. For example, when Medicare announced its star ranking system for Medicare Advantage health plans, CQC immediately educated providers about the Medicare value-based payment formula for health plans and its effect on provider payments and offered improvement support for star measures.

At CQC's formation, all stakeholders—plans, providers and purchaser—focused on P4P metrics to improve care for commercial HMO patients, a unifying purpose. Since then, value-based payments have proliferated across all business lines and at all levels of the system—health plans, hospitals, provider groups and physicians—and so have the measure sets: Physician Quality Reporting System (PQRS), Medicare Advantage stars, Accountable Care Organization (ACO) measures for integrated delivery systems, and value-based purchasing (VBP) for hospitals and meaningful use.

CQC's value has always been based on its ability to help its stakeholders perform better on measures associated with value-based payments. However, the proliferation of value-based programs complicates the process of setting aims, making it more difficult to find a common set of measures upon which to build program aims. Metrics do not necessarily line up across Medicare, commercial and Medicaid insurers. This affects CQC's member health plans most. Health plan priorities are diverging from each other as they make different decisions about investing in certain business lines and not others: Medicare, commercial, Medicaid expansion or the public exchange. It is increasingly difficult to find common ground. There is always more improvement work to do than funding to do it, so trade-offs need to be made.

Because CQC's geographic accountability is so large—the state of California—scale and spread has been critical. Methodologically, CQC does the following:

CQC Aims from 2015–2018

- **Build capacity within organizations to address total cost of care:** The most important achievement would be to create a "playbook" with ordered steps of implementation for strategies to both diagnose and address drivers of total cost of care; then use the playbook to spread methods of managing total cost of care across provider organizations.

- **Improve chronic illness care for populations of patients where clinical quality scores are lowest:** The most important achievement would be to show substantial improvement in Medi-Cal clinical quality measures and related Medicare Advantage star measures across a general population of 3 million people.

- **Expand the availability of intensive outpatient management for people with multiple medically complex conditions:** The most important achievement would be to increase the number of provider organizations offering effective outpatient complex-care management programs.

- Documents effective practices by publishing change packages for each aim, updated after collaboratives are completed
- Disseminates effective practices by holding teleconferences and one-day events and working closely with partners
- Implements best practices by offering collaboratives, often multiple waves over three years (e.g., chronic care measures, patient experience ratings, re-admissions), to engage leadership teams in system change within their organizations

Partners play a central role in dissemination strategy. CQC intentionally builds partnerships with organizations that have strong relationships with leaders and organizations CQC seeks to influence. For example, CQC co-sponsored an event with the state association of physician groups and recently built partnerships with improvement organizations working in the safety net.

The business case for improvement needs to be made over and over again in response to changes in the marketplace. CQC can only stay relevant, and therefore financially viable, if it assists its stakeholders and responds to new improvement imperatives. The right governance structure has helped the program stay close to the market, and stay relevant.

A sustainable improvement program needs to find the right balance between setting short-term, easily measurable goals and goals that drive fundamental system change over a longer time frame. A governing body needs to hold frank discussions about these goals and come to agreement on a portfolio of improvement initiatives to set appropriate expectations.

When considering funding opportunities, a program also needs to balance "opportunism" and discipline. The governing body provides important guidance on whether a particular opportunity meaningfully advances CQC's aims, and, if so, what role CQC should play in collaborative ventures in California, as lead agency or as supporting agency.

For example, CQC pursued a Center for Medicare & Medicaid Innovation (CMMI) award to test models of care for medically complex patients but did not pursue a role to spread improvement in maternity care. In addition, relationships built with other improvement organizations serving on the steering committee eases potentially sensitive conversations when negotiating roles bidding on funding opportunities.

Conclusion

In these case studies it's clear that while there are similarities, there's not a singular approach to collaborative governance. The impetus for collaboration varies as well as the stakeholders who are included in governance.

Collaborative governance is an evolutionary process. When considering what a structure may look like, you should know that depending on the lifespan of the collaborative and its complexity, there will more than likely be changes in the governance composition.

Regardless of the impetus for collaboration, having a mechanism to prioritize resources, both human and financial, is critical. Scope creep is a natural part of any project, so it's important to have oversight that keeps the strategic goals in mind and assesses any change that impacts them.

Finally, if sustainability of the collaborative is a goal, a diverse set of funding sources is important. A diverse funding approach may take the form of a larger single source with additional smaller sources or a more-or-less equivalent group of funders. Attention to the questions outlined in this chapter will set a firm foundation for the collaborative.

[1] Kaluzny, A., & Zuckerman, H. (1992). Two Perspectives for Understanding Their Effects on Health Services. *Hosp. Health Serv Adm , 37* (4), 477-490.

[2] Winslow, R. (2010, Dec. 15). A Healthcare Dream Team on a Hunt for the Best Treatments. *WSJ Blogs* .

[3] Mattessich, P., Murray-Close, M., & Monsey, B. (2008). *Collaboration: What Makes It Work* (Second Edition ed.). St. Paul, MN: Fieldstone Alliance.

[4] McGraw, D., & Letter, A. Pathways to Success for Multi-Site Clinical Data Research, eGEMs. *1* (1).

[5] Priest, E., Klekar, C., Cantu, G., & Berryman, C. (2014). Developing Electronic Data Methods Infrastructure to Participate in Collaborative Research Networks, eGEMs. *2* (1).

[6] Tomek, I., Sabel, A., Froimson, M., Muschler, G., Jevsevar, D., Koenig, K., et al. (2012). A Collaborative of Leading Health Systems Finds Wide Variations in Total Knee Replacement Delivery and Takes Steps to Improve Value. *Health Affairs , 31* (6), 1329-38.

[7] Bennis, W., & Ward Biederman, P. (1997). *The Secrets of Creative Collaboration.* New York: Basic Books.

[8] Kohn, L., Corrigan, J., & Donaldson, M. (2000). *To Err Is Human: Building a Safer Health System.* Washington, D.C.: National Academy Press.

[9] *Crossing the Quality Chasm: A New Health System for the 21st Century.* (2001). Institute of Medicine, Washington, D.C.: National Academy Press.

[10] Berenholtz, S., Pronovost, P., Lipsett, P., & al., e. (2004). Eliminating catheter-related bloodstream infections in the intensive care unit. *Crit Care Med , 32*, 2014-20.

[11] Lipitz-Snyderman, A., Steinwachs, D., Needham, D., Colantuoni, E., Morlock, L., & Pronovost, P. (2011). Impact of a statewide intensive care unit quality improvement initiative on hospital mortality and length of stay: retrospectiv comparative analysis. *BMJ , 342:d219.*

[12] Wilson, K. (2015, Feb.). California Health Insurers: Brink of Change. *California Health Care Foundation* .

[13] *University of California Berkeley, HAAS School of Business.* (n.d.). Retrieved from RAND Health: http://www.iha.org/pdfs_documents/p4p_california/MY2003TransparencyReport.pdf

[14] *California Quality Collaborative - Steering Committee.* (n.d.). Retrieved from http://www.calquality.org/about/steering-committee

CHAPTER 6

Designing Interventions

By Michael P. Silver, MPH, Jane Brock, M.D., MSPH
and Brianna Gass, MPH

Introduction

A major role of any collaborative is to accelerate adoption of new innovations
and spread effective practices across participating organizations. As Rogers[1]
and others point out, the nature of the intervention impacts the ease of
diffusion. Some interventions are easier than others to adopt and spread for
reasons we'll discuss below.

This chapter provides a framework for collaborative design using a
systematic review of the causes of and the systems and processes that produce
performance gaps in the identified problem areas. It also offers a review of
task design, operator characteristics and resources to address the problems.

Adapting interventions based on local context is another concept gaining
importance. Some interventions are designed as "models" or "bundles,"
often using research to prove their success. Yet there's growing consensus
that complete fidelity to an intervention design may impede adoption under
certain circumstances. Although the science and our understanding of local
contextual issues is nascent, this chapter will also explore when and how to
consider adapting an existing model.

Purpose and Process

Collaboratives accelerate the pace of change in healthcare organizations by engaging participants in collective learning and dedicated action. One way collaboratives promote effective action is through strategies that enable participants to drive change for current and future initiatives. The design processes outlined in this chapter consider collaborative interventions and organizational capacity building.

Diagnostic Review of the Performance Gap

When a team is charged with designing collaboratives, some framing has already taken place. A problem or opportunity (performance gap) has been proposed, identified and named. There's some evidence that the gap matters and won't simply resolve itself. Closing this performance gap will become the aim.

Teams should conduct a thorough assessment of the evidence of a performance gap and the ability to close it, with a clear understanding of why the changes should be adopted. They should also ensure the promoted changes offer clear benefit to participating organizations. Depending on the collaborative goal, this might involve expert review of medical evidence. It should also evaluate whether the evidence is relevant in other areas. If there's insufficient evidence of a performance gap, teams might reconsider their collaborative topic or goal.

After establishing evidence of a meaningful performance gap, teams can conduct a diagnostic review informing all collaborative activities. It helps to answer questions ranging from, "Is this a topic suitable for a collaborative?" and, "What precisely are we seeking to change?" to, "How do we make the change?" This review should involve collaborative sponsors and leadership, patients and families, clinical subject-matter experts, work process and design subject-matter experts, and collaborative operational staff.

Field practitioners can be directly involved or their input can be sought through interview or focus groups. In some collaboratives, other organizations perform these activities or there's deep experience with a particular intervention. Under these circumstances, collaboratives should evaluate the applicability of previous work to their particular participants.

If teams find evidence of a performance gap, the question is, "Why aren't providers participating in the collaborative already acting on the evidence?" The answers (and you can expect to see multiple contributors) will help develop a "theory of the gap" that helps identify intervention diffusion barriers and facilitators; it will also point to systems to leverage strategies that form the basis for the collaborative.

The following are the elements of a performance gap theory:

What is the Performance Gap?

Begin with the gap you're given. For example, reducing mortality from severe sepsis and septic shock is a hot topic nationally. You should ask:

- How does this performance gap impact patients? This should be answered from the patients' perspective, in their language and in their terms, and it should include emotional impact.
- How do you know this isn't a self-correcting gap?
  - Have you identified a relatively new innovation that's already diffusing on its own?
  - Are changes in the payment environment providing the necessary push?
- What's the evidence of the magnitude and importance of the gap?
- What's the evidence that performance can be improved? For example, do you see "bright spots" or evidence-based practices of higher performance?

- How do you know this performance gap isn't a symptom of a deeper problem that should be the focus of the collaborative?

Clearly, if the mortality rate from sepsis for participants is much higher than best-in-class performance, the gap may be worth addressing. If you also find evidence that similar organizations reduced mortality with well-described and tested changes and the volume of sepsis at participants is high, you would proceed with further analysis.

What Causes the Performance Gap?

In this part of the review, you get insight into the barriers to the innovation. You can begin by developing an inventory of the critical decisions, actions or practices required for the change. Each critical action can be analyzed to identify key decision-makers or process owners. Review each action and determine what you know about each one and why it's being taken:

- Have the critical process or system change actions been taken? Why? Why not? Review the areas where the change is occurring and where it isn't. Consider the progression:
    - **Awareness:** Do the decision-makers or frontline staff know about the innovation, its advantages and importance, and its applicability to their circumstances?
    - **Acceptance:** Do the decision-makers or frontline staff support making this change?
    - **Action:** Have the decision-makers or frontline staff taken action or dedicated the resources required to make the change?
    - **Execution:** Are the actions that have been taken likely to be effective? Has the organization employed a sound process design and change management approach?

- What intervention characteristics, environmental context, or organizational features are associated with adoption and uptake?

What drivers, external to decision-makers, are promoting or inhibiting uptake? Why aren't external drivers producing the desired change? For example, you may find in the sepsis analysis that a major barrier is that there's no standardized process to screen for sepsis or to even perform initial sepsis laboratory testing in the emergency department.

The results of this diagnostic review should provide an explicit description of the nature, importance and causes of the performance gap. At this point teams will decide if their proposed goal is suited for a collaborative. If so, the diagnostic review begins to identify potential collaborative participants and intervention targets. The review results can form a foundation for collaborative messaging shared with a commitment to transparency and an intent to refine theories through critique.

Systems Design Review

The collaborative's aim is some desired future state. A theory for how to achieve this future state can be mapped to strategies that might include specific changes to tasks, work processes, team composition or roles, communication and coordination, technology implementation, information management, education and training, supervision and management, performance monitoring, organizational leadership and governance, and even public policy. Systems design review identifies promising intervention opportunities and redesign strategies.

Like the diagnostic review, the systems design review gathers multiple perspectives, including those of patients and families. Direct observation of care practices and pilot tests of change can augment the review. In the sepsis example, you would want to observe practices in the emergency department and perhaps the intensive care unit and laboratory, to gain insights from various clinicians.

The systems design review might already be constructed. For example, the Surviving Sepsis Campaign (www.survivingsepsis.org) has international experience implementing evidence-based practices. When designing a collaborative, previous experience in other settings is important to consider. Using successful implementation of a collaborative elsewhere supports local customization as needed. Some interventions require more customization than others (see the "Adapting Improvement Initiatives" section of this chapter), and systems design review may also help in those instances.

Study the "bright spots" where the change is already occurring and seek out and learn from other successes. The systems design review is always looking for specific actions and strategies that can close the identified performance gap.

Getting to the required level of concrete detail can be exceptionally challenging. Informants, proponents of the change, and bright-spot practitioners may see the identified practices as expressions of deeply held values. Closing the performance gap is a matter of doing the right thing for the patient, and remembering why we're here. These are important perspectives that will be useful in collaborative design. The systems design review also has to push deeper into how those values find expression in the design of clinical work processes (Figure 1).

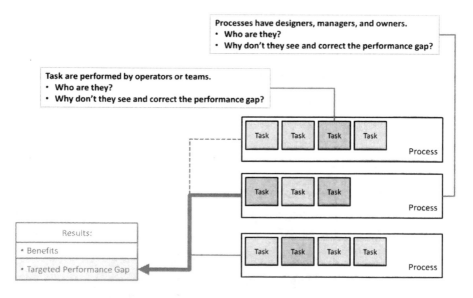

Figure 1. System design review

To aid in this review, teams can use analytic approaches such as process mapping[2], fault tree analysis, task analysis[3], cognitive task (decision) analysis[4] and applied behavior analysis[5] The process of such indepth review alone often leads to important insights. These insights, and not an expertly drawn process map, are the aims of this review. Teams can examine:

- **Leverage points created by common causal pathways:** These are places where the convergence of processes or concentrations of patients creates opportunities for effective design changes. The ideas of "trigger" and "capture" are two particular strategies to review. Look for how existing tasks or processes can be redesigned to set the desired actions in motion (trigger) or to intercept problems before they can have negative impact (capture). In the sepsis example, a trigger might be to order a lactate level anytime a blood culture is performed. Lactate levels above a threshold value trigger additional diagnostic or therapeutic actions.
- **Activate alternate resources:** Often at the leverage points, there are very busy people pursuing important goals. Your topic may be competing for their time and attention. We can look for other resources that can serve to trigger actions or capture problems. These other resources might cue or prompt action by a designated decision maker, or they might reallocate tasks. Resources to consider include information technology, other members of the clinical team, or the patients or caregivers themselves. With sepsis, the question arises whether the electronic medical record perform the screening instead of clinicians?
- **Differentiate:** It may be difficult to distinguish what causes bright spots to occur. To get at these differences, review teams can do the following:
  - Work with informants to define terms and process steps, actions and tasks in concrete detail.
  - Be sure to include review team members from outside of the collaborative focus area—even from outside of healthcare.

- Be prepared to augment the collection of review data with site visits that include direct observation of key tasks and processes.

- **Consider human factors[6,7] and behavioral drivers[8]:** Include a basic review of the possible intentions, distractions and motivations. For each of the critical tasks and operators identified, assess the following:
  - **Knowledge and intention:** Does the operator know the correct action, the situations in which it applies and their responsibility for the action? Do they intend to complete the expected action—in all applicable circumstances? Is the expected action compatible with the operator's current mental model (i.e., do they believe this is the correct action)?
  - **Attention management:** Is the operator likely to be distracted at critical junctures? Does the action require some vigilance on the part of the operator? Is this a "secondary" task—added on to another workflow? Are reminders or cues presented to the operator?
  - **Goal conflict:** Does the operator experience negative consequences for following the expected action? Does some other course of action save time? Might the operator experience a negative response from peers, coworkers, patients or family members? Is there something in the work environment that reinforces undesired behavior?

Key tasks or processes may be far removed from where the performance gap is observed.

Now you're ready to turn to intervention design.

Intervention Design

Some collaboratives create "driver diagrams" that explicitly state the necessary actions to drive activities to reduce the performance gap. Driver diagrams create a cascade of secondary drivers that promote primary drivers that lead to the change desired. During the systems design review, undoubtedly you established the linkage among many drivers. While driver diagrams are beyond the scope of this chapter, more information can be found at the NHS Institute for Innovation and Improvement[9] or the institute for Healthcare Improvement[10].

Collaborative design should recognize that no matter how important the proposed aim is, it's unlikely to be the only goal that the system or organization is pursuing. You should consider the potential for collaborative activities to conflict with other organizational goals. This goes beyond just avoiding collaboratives that could bankrupt participating organizations. Collaborative design should actively seek alignment with the other goals.

Almost every organization participating in a collaborative has a history and language of prior "flavor of the month" programs. Collaborative design also needs to be concerned about potential negative impact at the task level and disruptions to workflow, and concerned about the capacity for organizations to take on improvement initiatives and the energy these organizations are willing to devote to this topic.

In developing intervention designs, teams may consider the following strategies:

Strategy 1: Advance Broader System Goals

This approach goes beyond demonstrating that the collaborative aims are generally good for the organization or that they make some direct contribution to identified goals. Rather, this approach prioritizes intervention strategies based not only on their expected impact on collaborative aims but on their expected impact on overall system goals. This approach might narrow the collaborative focus to tasks or processes that not only impact collaborative aims but also many other patients. It can also be used to deliberately expand the scope of collaborative activities, to produce sustainable results or become an investment in organizational capacity for continuous improvement. Here are some thoughts about addressing multiple interventions.

Challenge: Addressing Multiple Interventions

Imagine that you've identified a task critical to the healthcare collaborative aim. You've discovered that in the course of busy clinical operations, it's a task sometimes overlooked or forgotten. You might propose a way to double-check for it, a reminder, or even an alarm with a flashing light and an annoying beep. This may address the problem, for a while. But you know how this ends: After a few years, every project team that comes along adds another alarm. They're all annoying and they're all ignored.

The identified problem was only a symptom, and a Band-Aid solution was applied. Instead, you can ask, "If our task is being omitted, what else is going on?" This sort of analysis might suggest focusing on reliability of specific tasks and processes (e.g., using a well-designed checklist or instituting a team briefing), with collaborative aims being advanced along with other organizational goals.

Following this strategy, you might identify four or five critical tasks or processes that are distributed in different operational areas throughout an organization. Each of these critical tasks impacts the collaborative aims and other important organizational goals

In our sepsis example, we found there was no process for screening and learned that other organizations have programed their electronic medical records (EMRs) to do real-time screening and create sepsis alerts. The IT department also has other requests to create EMR alerts, each valuable but cumulatively problematic. We don't want to overwhelm the staff with numerous alerts and the team looks at all of these situations to provide guidance.

Strategy 2: Leverage, Options and Progression

The systems design review should identify a number of potential approaches for closing the targeted performance gap. For some promising approaches, there may be variable or conflicting evidence of efficacy, with some sense that efficacy is sensitive to contextual factors. There may also be a variety of organizations in the collaborative to engage, all with variable resources, capacities, readiness and commitment to change, process design characteristics and prior experience with the collaborative targets.

The collaborative design team can help connect systems design review findings to participant action by developing an implementation guide. Such a guide could include the following:

- Detailed driver diagram or logic model
- Self-assessment with important organizational and contextual features identified in the diagnostic and systems design reviews
- Process for selecting and prioritizing promising approaches based on self-assessment findings
- Action plan for each promising approach featured:
  - Description of the process or task design change (and important variant options) or sequence of design changes
  - Description of the design principles employed
  - Implementation plan, resources required, operational areas and processes impacted
  - Measurement plan, including implementation milestones, process measures, outcomes and balancing measures
  - Anticipation of potential barriers and tips on how to overcome them, using the diagnostic and system design reviews or previous implementation efforts if available

Strategy 3: Resource Management

Teams designing collaborative interventions can expect that all the systems, organizations and operational areas they're working with will likely be seen as resource-constrained by their managers and leadership.

Resource management considerations not only impact collaborative participation and designs. When collaboratives recommend design changes that include committing to additional resources, especially on an ongoing basis, design teams should articulate the decision pathways organizations might take:

- **The intervention pays for itself:** It directly reduces overall production costs, risk and loss, waste or work. If this pathway is proposed, it may be necessary to articulate types of reduced costs and a plan for reclaiming avoided costs.
- **The intervention provides collateral benefits that sufficiently offset the costs:** An operational challenge associated with this pathway is that the collateral benefits are often not localized or accrue to another department's budget.
- **The intervention adds to production costs or requires additional resources:** This benefits patients because leadership will prioritize it over other organizational goals or commit resources without specifying where those resources will inevitably come from.

Ignoring resource management can affect sustainability so that when new topics, priorities or mandates need resources, organizations are unable to provide them.

Even with the thorough diagnostic review and planning detailed above, the actual success of the collaborative is dependent upon the success of implementing key processes performed at the participating organizations. Successful implementation often requires local adaptation, but how much and what kinds of adaptation will produce the desired outcome?

Adapting Improvement Initiatives

Most collaboratives designed to improve quality begin with at least one evidence-based model, which to most means a set of activities or components that have been tested as a bundle using research methods, associated with statistically significant outcomes and published in the peer-reviewed literature.

For purists, this means models that have shown efficacy through a randomized clinical trial. However, adaptation of research-established interventions during implementation is very common[11] and may enhance success, as non-adaptable programs imported from an external source that are not sensitive to local contexts and culture are less likely to be effective or sustained[12].

For example, more than 50 acute care providers joined forces with a local hospital in one community in an effort to improve care transitions. They determined that information transfer between the hospital and downstream providers was a root cause of readmissions and decided to implement a Universal Transfer Form to standardize the transfer of necessary patient information from one care setting to another. Shortly after they made this decision, the hospital implemented an EMR. This made the use of a paper-based form impractical, so the group decided to adapt information transfer practices to work electronically. The coalition regularly seeks feedback from clinical and administrative staff in the hospital and SNFs to identify the optimal content of information to be transferred when a patient discharges from the hospital.

As this example illustrates, each healthcare setting, system or community is unique. This makes adaptation of multi-component models or individual components, or mixing components from several different models, more the norm than the exception.

Adaptation Strategies

The following are common factors leading to deliberate or inadvertent adaptation strategies:

Limited Resources

Funding, staff time, availability of staff with necessary expertise, equipment and physical space are some resources that, if insufficient, may lead to reducing or eliminating components of a program. Ideally, less resource-intensive processes can be put in place to achieve the intended goals.

Structural Constraints in Existing Systems

It's often easier to modify a new model's structure than to change a process that has been in place and works well for a busy hospital unit or clinician.

For example, a hospital system in the South implemented a bundle of interventions aimed at earlier identification and prevention of delirium among older patients. It had originally planned to provide education to physicians about medications that increase the risk of developing delirium, but ultimately decided to remove these medications from automated order sets in the EMR or alert the physician to consider alternatives to high-risk medications. Physicians received education related to the rationale for these changes, but the changes to the order sets and prompts forced more widespread changes in practice than would have been possible through education alone.

Environmental Factors

Geography or demographic characteristics of the target population are often beyond the control of program planners. For instance, interventions that include a home visit may be unfeasible for programs serving large rural areas. In this case, planners may consider providing services via telephone or videoconference.

Concurrent or Parallel Programs

If components of an intervention package are already being provided elsewhere, they can be dropped from the new program, freeing resources to be invested in other components.

Involvement of Key Partners

Collaboratives that rely on participation of specific stakeholders for successful implementation may have to adapt by beginning the program with the components under the control of active participants while continuing to work on engagement of others.

For example, a community in the Southwest determined poor medication management to be a major factor in hospital readmissions and sought to implement medication management and reconciliation in an effort to reduce readmissions. Unfortunately, they were unable to proceed with this due to a lack of involvement among pharmacy stakeholders in their coalition. The community decided to move forward with interventions that addressed other causes of readmissions, while continuing the effort to engage pharmacists in the coalition.

Successful Adaptation

Despite being a common component of improvement initiatives, best methods for successful adaptation are not completely understood. This is, in part, due to a lack of established theoretical frameworks for studying them[13,14] and, in part, because we don't commonly use standardized tools to assess local culture and context despite the increasingly acknowledged influence of these elements[15]. Evidence suggests that adaptations are most successful when framed as modifications of core components in an evidence-based model, not as omissions.[16] The definitions of the core components of many complex cross-setting improvement models are still evolving.

It's therefore essential for collaborative teams to use strategies to balance the need to modify interventions with the potential of those modifications to weaken the impact of a thoroughly tested model:

- Begin a collaborative with a formal root-cause analysis to accurately identify major factors underlying the problem in the existing environment. Select interventions based on evidence that they are likely to impact the root cause, and minimize changing key elements directed at the root cause. If modifications require significant changes to elements that affect root cause, you should consider alternative strategies for addressing the problem.

- Review the literature for guidance about modification. Increasingly, models are being expressed as core versus modifiable components, and model developers and implementation teams are publishing results of testing modifications.
- Perform ongoing measurement of processes and interim progress to quickly detect whether adaptation is needed and whether the adaptation is likely to produce desired outcomes.
- Acknowledge that improvement is a dynamic and iterative process that can respond to changing realities. Improvement teams may need to weigh whether it's acceptable to reduce a component, with the associated loss of impact, or to mitigate it by other activities. The sacrifice may be worth the financial savings or other resources that will become available as a result of the adaptation.
- Anticipate barriers and brainstorm ways to address them during the planning phase. When working across care settings, partners will be familiar with their own settings and have prior experience with implementing new processes and making change within their organizations. The team can take advantage of this knowledge to anticipate adaptations.

For example, two health systems in different parts of the country implemented an electronic ICU (eICU) program to remotely monitor patients in rural hospitals. Both programs sought feedback from clinicians on the floors and in the monitoring unit and found a high degree of variation in attending physicians' willingness to allow the eICU to make care decisions. This made nurses uncomfortable calling the eICU for a consultation, decreasing their willingness to get help in situations that required it. Each hospital system addressed this problem differently. One simply mandated all consultations go through the eICU when the attending physician was not physically present in the unit. The other implemented and posted a rating system for physicians to designate which situations were acceptable for calling the eICU about their patient.

Both hospitals found their solutions to be effective, operationally and politically.

Collaborative teams should also recognize that adaptation is not limited to the planning phase of an intervention. Indeed, some of the most necessary modifications will be a result of challenges or barriers that emerge during implementation. Organizational culture is a critical factor that is often difficult to assess or know the impact of ahead of implementation but may ultimately force significant changes to be made for an intervention to be a good fit for the setting.

Conclusion

To paraphrase scientist Louis Pasteur, fortune favors the prepared team. This chapter proposes analysis and review processes by which the collaborative intervention design team can prepare itself, as well as testing adaptations that may accelerate adoption in different environments both to advance collaborative aims and to create meaningful professional development experiences for participants.

[1] Rogers, E. (2003). Diffusion of Innovations. *New York, Free Press.*

[2] Dettmer, H. (1997). *Goldratt's Theory of Constraints: A Systems Approach to Continuous Improvement.* Milwaukee, WI: ASQ Quality Press.

[3] Kirwan, B., & Ainsworth, L. (1992). *A Guide to Task Analysis.* Philadephia, PA: Taylor & Francis.

[4] Klein, G. (2004). *The Power of Intuition.* New York: Currency Doubleday.

[5] Krause, T. (1997). *The Behavior-Based Safety Process* (2nd Edition ed.). New York: Van Nostrand Reinhold.

[6] Norman, D. (1988). *Design of Everyday Things.* New York: Doubleday.

[7] Vincente, K. (2003). *The Human Factor: Revolutionizing the Way People Live with Technology.* . New York: Routledge.

[8] Mager, R., & Pipe, P. (1997). *Analyzing Performance Problems or You Really Oughta Wanna* (3rd Edition ed.). Atlanta, GA: CEP Press.

[9] *NHS Institute for Innovation and Improvement.* Retrieved from http://www. institute.nhs.uk/

[10] *Institute for Healthcare Improvement.* Retrieved from http://www.ihi.org/Pages/default.aspx

[11] Moulding, N., Silagy, C., & DP, W. (1999). A framework for effective managment of change in clinical practice: dissemination and implementation of clinical practice guidelines. *Am J Public Health , 8* (3), 177-183.

[12] Glasgow, R., Lichtenstein, E., & Marcus, A. (2003). Why don't we see more translation of health promotion research to practice? Rethinking the efficacy-to-effectiveness transition. *Am J Public , 93* (8), 1261-1267.

[13] Dy, S., Ashok, M., Wines, R., & Rojas Smith, L. (2015). A framework to guide implementation research for care transitions interventions. *Jounral for Healthcare Quality , 37* (1), 41-54.

[14] Nilsen, P. (2015). Making sense of implementation theories, models and frameworks. *Implementation Science , 10* (53).

[15] Balasubramanian, B., Cohen, D., Davis, M., Gunn, R., Dickinson, M., Miller, W., et al. (2015). Learning evaluation: blending quality improvement and implementation research methods to study healthcare innovations. *Implementation Science , 10* (31). p2.

[16] Kilbourne, A., Neumann, M., Pincus, H., & al, e. (2007). Implementing evidence-based interventions in health care: application of the replicating effective programs framework. *Implementation Science , 2* (1), 42, 4-5.

CHAPTER 7

Recruiting Participants, Strengthening Commitment

By By Elizabeth (Betsy) A. Lee, MSPH, BSN,
RN and Ken Alexander, MS, RRT
Wisconsin Collaborative for Healthcare Quality
(WCHQ) by Christopher Queram, MA
Using Progressive Cohorts by Alison L. Hong,
M.D. and Mary Reich Cooper, M.D., J.D.
Work with the Willing by Kevin O'Connor

Case Study: Wisconsin Collaborative for Healthcare Quality (WCHQ)

By Christopher Queram, MA

The growing acceptance of performance transparency among health systems is the result of achievements by organizations such as Wisconsin Collaborative for Healthcare Quality (WCHQ). Founded in 2003, WCHQ, commonly called "the Collaborative," is a voluntary non-profit (501c3) multi-stakeholder consortium of organizations committed to using publicly reported performance measures to help improve healthcare and the health status of people living in Wisconsin. In addition, WCHQ designs and facilitates collaborative learning sessions for sharing "best practices" among physicians. An integral part of the healthcare quality ecosystem within Wisconsin, WCHQ claims 40 healthcare provider organizations as members.

The Collaborative was formed as the result of two, separate dynamics that converged in a manner that laid the foundation for long-term success. The first of these was a desire on the part of the physician leaders from a number of Wisconsin's prominent integrated health systems to devise a method of measuring the performance of their medical groups on the basis of an entire population of patients irrespective of payment source. While acknowledged to be technically feasible, the health system leaders recognized that this "post-HEDIS" unit of analysis would gain added stature and credibility if it had the support of the business community.

About this same time, the second dynamic had emerged with the decision of The Alliance, a Madison-based employer cooperative to publish a "report card" on the performance of approximately 20 hospitals in southern Wisconsin. This action demonstrated that employers were serious about transparency, and galvanized the desire of the health system leaders to extend an invitation to representatives of the business community to join together in pursuit of a model that both could support.[1]

The Collaborative has received national recognition for its work and has made numerous contributions to the emerging evidence base on the science of measurement and reporting. Peer-reviewed research, as well as measures reported on the WCHQ website (http://www.wchq.org), show that WCHQ has played a significant role in the improvement in quality among the physician groups in Wisconsin[2] and the quality of performance over time.[3]

WCHQ's goals to advance the quality and affordability of healthcare and the overall health of the population are at the vanguard of organizations emerging at the community, regional and state levels. These "regional health improvement collaboratives" (RHICs) share a number of common characteristics:

- Non-profit status

- Multi-stakeholder governance (typically consisting of provider organizations, health plans/payers, purchasers and consumer advocacy groups)

- Active engagement of public sector agencies (Medicaid, public health and state employee purchasing agencies)

- Focus on performance measurement/public reporting and performance improvement

- Relatively unstable funding streams, typically consisting of membership dues, foundation grants, public sector appropriations and contracted services

While RHICs pursue broadly similar work, their distinctive characteristics are a reflection of the unique environment in which they operate. In the case of WCHQ, several factors have shaped the organization's evolution into an integral part of the healthcare quality ecosystem within Wisconsin. In a very real sense, these factors work together to create the platform needed for the long-term sustainability of quality healthcare.

Voluntary Participation

The Wisconsin Legislature has been known to largely eschew the enactment of healthcare mandates since the late 1990s individual assessment. Rather than seeking to change this long-standing political orthodoxy, the Collaborative has embraced it; indeed, the Collaborative operates with the philosophy that while mandates can compel participation, they cannot assure commitment. In a very real sense, WCHQ seeks to use this to its advantage by developing, implementing and relentlessly focusing its voluntary model on two goals designed to bring tangible and concrete benefits to its members: generating and reporting valid, reliable and actionable comparative performance metrics and convening and facilitating collaborative learning sessions.

This clarity of mission and purpose, as well as essential quality customer service, has helped to grow the Collaborative's membership from nine organizations to 40 since its beginning. Under its by-laws, organizations eligible for membership are those who provide ambulatory healthcare services and for whom performance can be reported. The Collaborative's membership includes free-standing multi-specialty group practices, hospitals, single specialty primary care practices, health plans and integrated health systems.

Guiding Principles and Values

Before the reaching the decision to incorporate the Collaborative as a legal entity, leaders from a number of Wisconsin's large health systems—along with employers, purchaser coalitions and consumer organizations, collectively referred to as "business partners"—spent close to a year working together to build a common understanding of each other's motivations and goals around performance measurement and reporting. By taking time to share with one another their hopes, fears, aspirations and anxieties surrounding the growing push for greater transparency, the participants gradually began to move forward together. The leaders knew that the success of the organization depended on the ability to maintain the trust and commitment forged during this formative period. This led the group to adopt a set of values that include trust, participation, inclusiveness, shared responsibility, openness, adaptive self-governance, intellectual output, acknowledgement and transparency, all of which the Collaborative operates by to this day.

Mission

The growing acceptance of performance measurement has led to an explosion of demands from both the public and private sectors. Data demands can be linked to a variety of initiatives—health plan reporting requirements, employer initiatives (Leapfrog), public sector purchasers (Medicaid as well as the various Centers for Medicare and Medicaid Services (CMS) initiative such as 1 Million Hearts, the Hospital Engagement Network (HEN), Physician Quality Reporting System (PQRS), Meaningful Use (MU) and the Value modifier), professional societies (Maintenance of Certification (MOC), Performance Improvement - Continuing Medical Education (PI-CME), "Get with the Guidelines") and regulators (Joint Commission core measure requirements). This accentuates the importance of maintaining an organization of committed volunteers such as the Collaborative, which uses its social capital and trust in its members and stakeholders, along with its guiding principles and values, to support its vision.

The tension around measurement burden is harnessed to positive effect through an ongoing and iterative process designed to ensure that the Collaborative's measure portfolio achieves a balance between core measures promulgated at a national level (for example, by CMS through its mandated reporting programs such as PQRS and Meaningful Use) and those that reflect the priorities and interests of Wisconsin stakeholders.

The Collaborative also seeks to simplify and streamline the data-submission process. For example, it has built a clinical data repository for member organizations to submit large patient-level data files from their billing and clinical record systems to be used to develop performance measurement metrics and reports that are widely recognized for their validity, reliability and actionability. This repository is unique among regional collaboratives nationally and allowed WCHQ to pursue designation by Centers for Medicare & Medicaid Services (CMS) as a qualified clinical data registry (QCDR) in which it can submit data under various federal reporting programs (e.g., Physician Quality Reporting System, Meaningful Use). In addition, WCHQ's collaborative learning sessions, geared toward practice transformation, revolve around the sharing of best practices in a noncompetitive way.

Introduction

Even with an optimal design and a compelling aim for improvement, a collaborative will never succeed without a committed and engaged group of participants. It's not enough to recruit organizations to join the effort; collaboratives must recruit organizations whose leaders commit to participate wholeheartedly with conviction, energy and a spirit of sharing.

Examples of large numbers of committed participants that have made broad-scale improvements include the Centers for Medicare and Medicaid Services (CMS) Partnership for Patients initiative launched in 2011. This collaborative works to improve the quality, safety and affordability of healthcare, along with other national, state and regional collaboratives tackling specific healthcare improvement topics.[4]

A successful collaborative recruitment strategy relies not only on the strength of the design and underlying aim of the initiative, but also on the depth of trust that potential participants hold in the organizing entity and the abilities of that group to provide both structure and flexibility throughout the process. Three key factors can contribute to robust recruitment and enduring engagement, whether the collaborative is focused on internal system improvement or broad-scale local, state, regional or national efforts:

1. Create a sound recruitment plan linked to a strong collaborative *design and a strong support infrastructure*
2. *Engage stakeholders and partners,* strengthened by existing relationships and a commitment to jointly develop a strong value proposition and a vision of better healthcare
3. Develop a *network of champions* within and between participating organizations
4. Plan for ongoing recruitment and commitment

Whether organizing a collaborative focused on one topic or a complex network of topics, the singular most important element for successful recruitment is establishing a compelling purpose for the collaborative. Bold aims for change with achievable, finite numeric targets provide the basis for the story of why people and organizations would want to join a collaborative effort. It's not enough to build the collaborative design only around "what" needs to be improved, but "how" to achieve the aims (the improvement knowledge) is also necessary.[5] While these elements are critical, true commitment happens only when people fully understand "why" joining a collaborative improvement effort will advance their learning and action toward specific aims.[6,7] What really matters is engaging a broad audience with a common will for change, ideas for improvement and a commitment to execute it, and then providing the infrastructure and support to enable them to do the work.[8]

Recruitment and ongoing retention planning begin in advance of the quality improvement collaborative (QIC) launch and extend throughout the spread period. Key recruitment phases and engagement activities include the following.

Inspire Initial Enrollment and Commitment

While a bold aim such as Partnership for Patients' goal to reduce preventable hospital-acquired conditions and hospital readmissions may inspire people to join an initiative, the details about how participating organizations will commit to work together and participate in data submission and reporting are equally vital. Some collaborative designers require participants to sign a commitment form detailing the activities and expectations of participants, along with the resources the organizing entity will provide.

Setting and describing clear expectations during recruitment will assist with enrollment. Participants want to know not only what will be expected of their teams, but also how the collaborative will help them achieve their organizations' strategic aims. Clear and concise communication regarding data collection and submission requirements, intermediate and long-term outcome targets, and collaborative learning timelines will increase the chances for broad organizational engagement.

Address Variation and Staging

Most collaborative learning and improvement networks feature voluntary participation, whether through a fee-based participation model, grant supported involvement or coalition-based engagement. When the collaborative focus is to engage as many participants as possible to achieve broad spread, the likelihood exists for great variation in improvement capacity at the level of the participating organizations. In designing large-scale collaborations, this presents a challenge related to where to set the minimum participation requirements. If the barrier to entry is low (small or waived participation fee, minimal data submission requirement, low reporting requirements), organizations may initially commit with a "wait and see" attitude until they understand the relative benefit they might gain. Conversely, if participants perceive the level of effort and cost to be too high relative to the anticipated outcomes for their organization, the collaborative organizers may discover challenges in recruitment and retention of participants.

Successful recruitment plans address such barriers during the planning phase. It's critical to identify mechanisms to reduce the burden of paperwork, simplify and align measurement strategies, and minimize travel and time away from the home organization. This plan should also outline any options to join at different levels or staged time periods to accommodate varying degrees of readiness for change.

For instance, some organizations may be able and willing to begin with first-order changes or aims but don't feel ready to address complex changes due to competing priorities or other challenges. These reluctant organizations may be willing to join through a cohort design or phased-in approach. Allowing for this type of staged entry will provide greater incentives for the late adopters to join and begin learning from their peers and faculty.

Using Progressive Cohorts

By Alison L. Hong, M.D. and Mary Reich Cooper, M.D., J.D.

When one of the largest hospitals in Connecticut was unable to decrease its adverse event incidence despite using national best practices, it joined a cohort of the Connecticut Hospital Association, a state high-reliability collaborative (HRC) that was started three years earlier. After joining the cohort, the hospital's rate of reported near misses is up, its Serious Safety Event Rate is down, and employees say the hospital has changed the way it conducts business.[9] How did these results happen?

The Connecticut Hospital Association applies a progressive cohort model, allowing hospitals the flexibility to participate when they are optimally prepared. Collaborative cohorts, known to be successful in reducing the spread of healthcare-associated infection,[10] move organizations through training and measurement together, supporting peer-to-peer learning and economies of scale, without requiring all members of the collaborative to be at the same point in implementation. The cohort size and the resources provided to support it are determined by the collaborative's accelerator, a person or group that pushes change forward using the science of innovation and the dynamics of the cohort.

Work with the Willing

By Kevin O'Connor

I learned a valuable lesson while preparing for my first collaborative learning session when I realized a substantial number of hospitals weren't planning to participate. I became concerned that we wouldn't be able to make meaningful progress, so I asked my co-director what we should do. His reply was as wise as it was brief. He said, "We don't need to be concerned with them; we just need to focus on those who want to participate. The others will come along when it's right for them to join in." Within two years, the participation rate more than doubled.

There may be a spectrum of engagement, especially in the early stages, with some not engaged nor willing to do the necessary work. This may be exacerbated by the fact that, in general, the benefit to the participants is directly proportional to the effort put in. Not surprisingly, the most actively engaged will derive the most benefit, and the least actively engaged will derive the least benefit.

It's always worth the effort to understand the reasons why some choose to be less engaged than others, and to attempt to help them to become more active participants. However, there's a substantial opportunity cost associated with this. Early improvements in outcomes tend to create a snowball effect, inspiring more and more participants to increase their level of participation, which in turn generates even greater improvement in outcomes. Therefore, working with the willing, especially in the early stages, is a sound strategy for success.

Using a cohorting approach to implement HRC principles makes sense because organizational readiness is a critical component to success, and it may take one to two years to prepare for high reliability.[11] High reliability supports a teamwork-based safety culture so inevitable human mistakes don't lead to patient harm. This methodology emphasizes inter-professional interventions, behavioral changes, structured leadership and culture shifts, particularly toward a culture of safety as a core value.[12]

Changing the culture of safety gives the participants purpose; they're saving lives. Their motives could be altruistic or economic, but because of the cohort approach, there are like-minded individuals at a number great enough to be a critical mass. Implementing a collaborative statewide allows healthcare organizations to exchange staff and doctors as well as ideas, knowing that each organization is trained with the same methodology.

You can expedite and enhance enrollment through early recruitment of high performers or known innovators on the topic, as well as organizations with a history of early adoption. Obtaining commitment from diverse stakeholders with deep content knowledge will also increase the likelihood that other organizations will participate. Strategies for success in building momentum in the recruitment phase include targeting leaders in health systems, regions, and influential groups and associations. Linking associations and other professional groups will not only assist in recruitment for a specific collaborative topic, but also eventually serve as the building blocks for a sustainable infrastructure for change and improvement.

Plan a Sustainable Infrastructure

Creating an enduring infrastructure for building improvement capacity at a local, state, regional or national level relies on building trust and fostering relationships with key stakeholders and experienced improvement experts. You can develop networks based upon geographic areas or common interests. You can then use regionalized models or affinity groups as building blocks for expansion across states, nations or content communities.

An example of a functional statewide infrastructure is the network of 11 regional patient safety coalitions in Indiana, fostered by the Indiana Hospital Association (IHA) during 2007-2011 to promote spread of patient safety and quality improvement throughout the state. IHA leveraged the efforts of existing regional patient safety coalitions, particularly the Indianapolis Coalition for Patient Safety. Formed in 2003, The Indianapolis Coalition for Patient Safety, Inc. (ICPS) provides a forum for area hospitals to share information about best practices and work together to solve patient safety issues. Membership is comprised of all six health systems in the city with a shared vision to make central Indiana the safest place to receive healthcare in the nation.

According to ICPS president, James Fuller, Pharm.D., "It's a unique model, where health system leadership, as well as front line staff, undertake projects that use evidence-based, patient-centered strategies to achieve a standardized approach to patient care, accelerating improvements in patient safety across the community. These organizations have come together, and while competitors in the market place, have agreed not to compete on safety. This makes Indianapolis health systems uniquely positioned to continue to improve patient outcomes and reduce harm."

A reliable infrastructure for change and improvement balances coordination and segmentation. A strong organizing entity features both centralized and decentralized functions. While there's an element of the support that can be centralized, an organic infrastructure with multiple loci of control in decentralized groups or coalitions creates a network of support for ongoing efforts and strengthened local relationships. As much as possible, collaborative organizing groups should focus on developing disseminated improvement capacity as a platform for future improvement collaboration. A coalition-based model allows for diverse stakeholders to work together over time, building trust and local capacity to respond to new or emerging issues.

Develop an Agile, Transparent Operations Team

The nature of a thriving learning and improvement collaborative is that the community of practice informs the work and changes the conversation about the topic during the course of the initiative. The new learning comes from successful tests of change at the local organization level, so an organizing entity is constantly adapting to the new knowledge and changing needs. This fosters the climate for ongoing recruitment to engage in sequential collaborative improvement topics. The QIC organizing team can create momentum and energy by providing opportunities for participants to learn from successful peer leaders and organizations. The value of sharing both successes and challenges with peers cannot be overstated. The essence and strength of an improvement collaborative is found in the numerous examples of successful tests of change spreading throughout the learning community. In a truly sustainable framework for collective change, the web of relationships among individual participants and stakeholders will develop to the point that the original collaborative organizer may eventually serve only in a facilitative and convening role.

A key role of a flexible operational team is to match the need for regular communication with appropriate message, pace and volume of information. Messaging that ensures everyone receives the same information in a timely, consistent manner, that is customized to varying levels of interest and involvement, is crucial. Not only does this ensure that all stakeholders are informed, but also increases the likelihood that they will be engaged in what's happening at their organizations.

Engage Leaders, Stakeholders and Partners

The single biggest factor when engaging an organization's leadership is simply gaining their attention, which is usually extremely challenging given the many pressures and competition for their time and energy. A successful collaborative is impossible without full commitment of an organization's senior leadership, including its board and medical staff.

To engage leaders, it's important to first connect to what drives them and to an overarching purpose that has meaning to them. This means connecting the aim of the collaborative to the strategic goals and vision of the organizations, whether that's to reduce harm to patients, improve system results and efficiency, or improve an organization's reputation in the community. The more you understand the goals, needs and motivations of the leaders you're trying to engage, the better your chances of gaining their attention.

Face-to-face communication is an ideal mechanism for engaging leaders and garnering buy-in. If you're leading a collaborative, that could mean anything from providing formal updates at stakeholder meetings to providing quick tidbits of information to a senior leader about the progress of their organization. While the logistics behind planning and accomplishing meaningful face-to-face meetings can be challenging, if you're leading multiple organizations, whether regionally or statewide, the effectiveness and importance of sitting down with leadership as often as possible can greatly impact a project's success. It allows for relationship-building, more effective communication, the ability to understand and react to non-verbal communication, and additional opportunities to build trust. This also requires flexibility on the part of the operational team to "get out in the field" and may require coverage of a broad territory.

In crafting communications to senior leaders, finding the appropriate messenger matters greatly. Peer-to-peer communication is effective and powerful and can form the basis of a multi-prong approach to engagement.

The Louisiana Hospital Association's (LHA) Hospital Engagement Network, used such a strategy to promote widespread engagement in Partnership for Patients. The project director, a senior staffer and prior hospital CEO, approached the C-suite, board and medical staff. He successfully leveraged his relationships with senior leaders to communicate the project goals, needs, benefits and so on, to the audience with the highest level of influence within each organization. Simultaneously, the project manager approached the quality directors and mid-level managers with the same message. Staff improvement advisors communicated with line staff and supervisory-level leaders at each hospital.

Delivering a similar but tailored message in multiple "peer-to-peer" environments was extremely effective in reinforcing the salient points of the message to ensure that everyone was on the same page.

Once you have an audience with leadership and those with some level of influence, the message is extremely important. From one author's experience, regardless of who is delivering the message, the key to gaining buy-in and acceptance by leaders is to appeal to those aspects of the project that positively impact them or their organization's needs in a way that helps them connect to the purpose of the initiative.

For example, a financial executive is worried about the financial health of the organization, so approaching a need framed in a financially meaningful context will obviously have more impact than a purely clinical perspective. Not that CFOs don't care about patients or the care they receive, but their priority is to consider the financial implications of actions and decisions.

To amplify this point, consider this hypothetical example. Let's say the quality director and the case management director of an urban hospital want to implement a readmissions reduction initiative that involves hiring two full-time staff members. Their analysis shows they can cut their readmissions in half if they implement this one initiative. Their most recent readmission reduction program penalty percentage from the federal government, based on CMS' formula, is 1.75 percent, which translates to a $500,000 reduction in their Medicare payments over the course of the next federal fiscal year. By adding two staff members dedicated to reducing readmissions, at a total payroll cost of less than $120,000 per year for both employees, they can show the CFO that the cost benefit of absorbing additional staff dollars will result in mitigating future readmissions penalties, effectively recovering an additional $380,000 to the bottom line. The CFO is now paying attention. Demonstrating a sensitivity to the finances of the organization helps build awareness, acceptance, credibility and, perhaps most importantly, goodwill.

This premise holds regardless of the target audience. Physicians like to see processes that improve patient care, are simple to implement and that improve the efficiency of care delivery. Hospital boards want to see those things that play to the organizations' overall health, community perception and population health outcomes.

Communicating and managing the message in a way that stresses the target audience's priorities creates an attentive audience that will at least listen with interest to what's being communicated. And in instances where priorities differ between audiences, helping them understand each other's frames of reference and challenges can go a long way in promoting the value and necessity of supporting each other's needs. This helps build an important bridge for effective change.

Another way to engage leaders is to provide more formalized education to help them understand the need, process and methods associated with the improvement activity. The multi-tiered approach used by the LHA Hospital Engagement Network, mentioned previously, involved developing a presentation that not only described and articulated the initiative and its components and expectations but also provided background information that set the stage. The project director traveled across the state presenting to hospital boards, medical staff (both executive and general medical staff committees), senior leaders, management teams (mid-level) and staff-level individuals. They designed the presentation to provide a high-level overview of the project and its goals after clearly posing the case for change. It included a brief history of the major components of healthcare reform and the delivery system, national and state level issues, and how a pre-reform delivery system was set up to fail if not approached differently. After they established the case for change, they introduced the opportunity for collaboration, along with the necessary actions on the part of the organization to effectuate enrollment and subsequent meaningful change.

In this example, every level of the organization received a core message that was consistent and understandable. The actual slides used in the presentation were identical, regardless of audience, but the presenter used different examples and points of emphasis to ensure that everyone, regardless of rank, title or position in the organization, understood the important takeaways in a way that was relatable to them in their specific roles.

134

While standardized message delivery is sufficient in some cases, it's important to communicate potentially complex and easily misunderstood information in whatever manner necessary to ensure understanding and acceptance throughout an organization. This helps pave the way for senior leadership support and engagement.

Form a Network of Champions

In addition to developing connections with senior leaders, a successful ongoing recruitment and engagement strategy includes a direct effort to network with improvement teams at each participating organization. These teams are composed of frontline clinical staff, as well as quality improvement directors and support personnel. Connecting with the implementation team and key clinical leaders throughout each organization, as well as in designated regions or affinity groups, will ensure the development of champions who can convey the importance of participation to their colleagues and peers, both within and outside their organizations.

It's often beneficial to frame the learning opportunities within the collaborative as an added bonus of professional development in the domains of system improvement, patient safety science, teamwork, inter-professional communication and high reliability. Creating personal and professional development opportunities for these champions and quality leaders will advance a broad-based workforce enhancement strategy in a state or region. Collaboratives offer individuals the chance to improve their competencies in delivering presentations, serving as coaches or peer mentors and evaluating evidence-based practice. This may enhance joy and meaning in work and offer potential career advancement.

A collaborative that focuses not only on the content of the improvement topic but also on the context of the community and the science of improvement will highlight opportunities for champions to lead. Expanded leadership competencies in communication and teamwork provide the platform for individual champions to participate in improvement teams with stakeholders from diverse community organizations. The inclusion of patients and family members in the collaborative advisory team and learning sessions offers additional venues for skill development related to the socioeconomic aspects of population health.

Conclusion

Recruitment and engagement success reach far beyond the initial collaborative planning activities. Successful programs plan ahead to leverage content-specific learning in a way that develops leader competencies across the continuum of participants—from the program organizers to the system leaders to the content and process champions. A commitment to fostering trust among diverse stakeholders and across multiple projects will enhance the chances of creating a long-term sustainable infrastructure for change and improvement.

Each leader's personal and professional journey toward transformational change requires a network of individuals and systems acting in support of not only the topic at hand, but also advancement of the science of improvement and the compelling reasons to act together to achieve a common bold aim.

[1] Hibbard, J., Stockard, J., & Tusler, M. (2005). Hospital Performance Reports: Impact On Quality, Market Share, and Reputation. *Health Affairs , 24* (4), 1150-1160.

[2] Smith, M., Wright, A., Queram, C., & Lamb, G. (2012). Public reporting helped drive quality improvement in outpatient diabetes care among Wisconsin physician groups. *Health Affairs , 31* (3), 570-77.

[3] Lamb, G., Smith, M., Weeks, W., & Queram, C. (2013). Publicly reported quality-of-care measures influenced Wisconsin physician groups to improve performance. *Health Affiars , 32* (3), 536-543.

[4] McCannon, J., & Berwick, D. (2011). A new frontier in patient safety. *JAMA , 305* (21), 2221-2222.

[5] Kilo, C. (1999). Improving care through collaboration. *Pediatrics , 103*, 383-93.

[6] Solberg, L. (2007). Improving medical practice: a conceptual frakework. *Ann Fam Med , 5* (3), 251-256.

[7] Bleser, W. (2014). Strategies for achieving whole-practice engagement and buy-in to the patient-centered medical home. *Ann Fam Med , 12* (1), 37-45.

[8] Nolan, T. (2007). Execution of Strategic Improvement Initiatives to Produce System-Level Results. *IHI Innovation Series white paper*. Cambridge, MA: Institute for Healthcare Improvement (Available on www.ihi.org)

[9] Throop, C., & Stockmeier, C. (2009). The HPI SEC & SSER Patient Safety Measurement System for Healthcare. *HPI White Paper Series* (1).

[10] Berenholtz, S., & al., e. (2011). Collaborative cohort study of an intervention to reduce ventilator-associated pneumonia in the intensive care unit. *Infect Control Hosp Epidemiol , 32* (4), 305-14.

[11] Smith, M. (2007). Disruptive innovation: Can healthcare learn from other industries? A conversation with Clayton M. Christensen. *Health Affairs , 26*, 288-95.

[12] Weick, K. (1987). Organizational culture as a source of high reliability. *29* (2), 112-28.

CHAPTER 8

Helping Participants Optimize Their Effectiveness

By Sarah M. Stout, MPAff

"Our team had an epiphany about a year into the CCTP Learning
Collaborative. We realized that we needed to stop thinking of PDSAs
as projects that we do along the side of running our program. We
need to infuse quality improvement throughout everything we
do—we need to run our program through PDSAs. That has been
a powerful shift in thinking and in how we run our program.
—Maria Basso-Lipani, Director, Preventable Admissions
Care Team, Mount Sinai Hospital, New York

Introduction

In 2012, the Centers for Medicare & Medicaid Services launched a multi-year collaborative for all communities participating in the Community-based Care Transitions Program (CCTP) to reduce 30-day hospital readmission rates for high-risk Medicare beneficiaries. Maria Basso-Lipani of the CCTP at Mount Sinai Hospital in New York and chair of the CCTP faculty reported having an epiphany about one year into the program when she realized that she needed to stop thinking about quality improvement (QI) work as something her team does in addition to running the program. Rather, they need to integrate QI methods and, specifically, plan-do-study-act (PDSA) methods into how she and her team run the program.

In a collaborative, participants are learning to produce results. The sponsor's role is to help them. Sponsors do this by creating a collaborative community that has a shared vision for improvement, a sense of urgency for achieving results, and a common commitment to using QI methods with rigor and discipline.

This chapter provides guidance about how collaborative sponsors can build a community that supports participants in making breakthroughs in performance. It focuses on 1) how to build the sense of community and trust necessary to achieve free and open exchange of ideas and 2) how to build participants' capacity with and commitment to QI methods, with the aim to transform how the participants approach their work, as with the Mount Sinai care transitions team.

Grow Peer-to-Peer Sharing

Collaboratives thrive on multi-directional learning, where participants learn from each other primarily and from the collaborative sponsors, external stakeholders and experts. Collaboratives are designed to facilitate the free and continuous exchange of ideas among participants. It is common for this sharing of ideas to grow over time as participants build relationships and confidence with each other and the sponsors.

Building trust in a collaborative requires understanding, a thoughtful approach and patience. This should be an explicit goal of collaborative activities, particularly in the beginning when participants and sponsors are still shaping and understanding the culture of the collaborative.

Promote Interaction

Probably the most critical ingredient to building trust is time. At the beginning of a collaborative, participants often feel they may not have a lot in common with other members. They tend to focus on how they're unique, with respect to their programs, organizations and operating environments. However, despite their differences, they're working toward a common purpose and will experience some of the same challenges and successes as other members.

In-person meetings early in the collaborative are highly desirable. Nothing creates trust and rapport more readily than face-to-face interactions, especially if time is built in for meaningful sharing and exchange among the participants. It's important to guide and structure sharing to focus on the implementation tactics that generate shared experience. In face-to-face meetings, participants are more likely to be vulnerable and ask for help with their challenges, which will build affinity among others with similar challenges.

If it's not possible to bring the participants together physically, provide opportunities to engage them virtually; though keep in mind that this will take longer to build rapport and confidence. Consider holding calls more frequently in the beginning to allow trust and fellowship to develop.

Intentionally Build Trust and Exchange Ideas

An effective tool that many successful collaboratives use to establish trust is the "Signature Style," which is a method for running calls, webinars and meetings. One of the key concepts underlying the style, "net-forward energy," is useful in creating an atmosphere of openness and assurance. Consider framing a learning event, particularly in the early stages of a collaborative, by acknowledging that the "energy in the room" is critical to the success of the event and requesting that participants be aware of how they think and speak so they're contributing to a net-forward rather than a net-backward energy.

When listening to each other's experiences in a collaborative setting, it's natural for participants to think about why other participants' knowledge isn't relevant to them or why their successful strategy or innovation wouldn't work for them. Perhaps they've tried it before and it was unsuccessful, or they think the other participants are too different from them for their experiences to have relevance.

A meeting achieves net-forward energy when the participants agree to set aside critical judgment and listen to each other for possibilities and opportunities. The application of net-forward energy can create positive feedback loops.

Make Sharing Data the Norm

When collaborative participants are willing to share their program data with each other, it's a strong sign of trust. Many organizations enter into collaboratives reluctant to share their data because they fear that their peers or a funder will judge them or they have concerns about sensitive data.

A collaborative, however, cannot thrive unless the members are willing to share their progress, including their data. The collaborative exists to support continuous improvement toward a common goal. Data is required to measure improvement, identify top performers, surface their emerging best practices and prioritize areas for action. The sponsor can help overcome barriers to sharing data in a number of ways:

- Ask permission
- Acknowledge and celebrate the sharing of lessons learned

- Demonstrate the value of data-sharing by making meaningful use of the data and reporting it back to the participants
- Start with data that participants feel more comfortable sharing
- Share aggregate or blinded data first, if necessary, until the participants are comfortable sharing their data

It may take time, attention and well-crafted messaging to achieve a collaborative culture where the participants trust each other and the sponsor enough to share their experiences and data, but it's well worth the effort. When that confidence is in place and collaborative members are sharing their knowledge—and their results—the collaborative becomes a powerful engine for change and improvement. When top performers share their emerging best practices, their results are what will capture the attention of and inspire to action the other collaboratives.

Create a Community Identity

Borrowing the words of educational theorist Etienne Wenger in describing communities of practice, a collaborative is a group of people "bound by what they do together ... solving difficult problems[1]." Wenger theorizes that a community of practice defines itself along three dimensions: what it's about, how it functions and what capabilities it has produced. This provides a useful framework for how to help a collaborative establish its identify.

Three elements are essential to defining a collaborative identity:

1. **What it's about: The aim:** The sponsor, in part, defines the collaborative identity and establishes the common goal, aim or "joint enterprise" that the participants will work toward, the time frame for achieving the goal, and the measures for success.

As the participants articulate the goal of the collaborative and put it in the context of their organizations and communities, the aim becomes a shared vision.

2. **How it functions: All teach, all learn:** The principles on which the collaborative operates also shape the community identity. Collaboratives usually operate on an "all teach, all learn"[2] principle, which differentiates collaboratives from other types of activities in which learning is didactic or one-way. In a collaborative, learning is multi-directional. All participants learn from each other, their sponsor and external stakeholders. Over time, participants develop a shared language and set of practices that define how they engage with each other. These practices and routines are the engine of the collaborative. They drive participants to share their lessons learned with each other, to process what they are learning from each other, and identify and prioritize action items for testing. This is a powerful function capable of producing remarkable results.

3. **What it produces: A body of knowledge about what works:** Collaboratives typically build on a body of knowledge about best practices that high-performing organizations have demonstrated to work. Collaboratives contribute to that body of knowledge by capturing and spreading new best practices as they emerge. A "change package," which provides the roadmap for achieving improvement, captures foundational and emerging best practices. It describes the strategies and drivers that are essential to change and provides a menu of testable actions that organizations and communities can choose from and prioritize when developing their improvement plans. A "driver diagram" is a complementary document that visually depicts the primary and secondary drivers and associated actions that will help participants achieve their aims.

Collaborative sponsors and participants will generate other materials, including collections of practices, resource guides, tools, videos, presentations and patient stories. All of this should be documented and exist as an archive for use beyond the duration of the collaborative.

Provide Technical Support

Collaboratives provide technical support to members to help them achieve success. Technical support comes in the form of shared learning about the details and the specifics of implementation, not broad theory or organizational design.

Promote an Exchange of Ideas

Peer-to-peer sharing should be part of every group interaction. Strategies for optimizing peer-to-peer exchange vary by type of event.

Facilitate Peer-to-Peer Exchange in Face-to-Face Meetings

Facilitating peer-to-peer exchange is relatively easy in face-to-face meetings by providing opportunities for organizations to interact through facilitated small group discussions, open spaces, networking sessions, poster sessions and informal exercises during plenary sessions. Each session of a face-to-face meeting should build in time for participants to talk with each other through guided exercise or information networking. Sessions dedicated to peer-to-peer exchange should be structured as small group discussions, poster sessions or informal networking exercises. Each of these modes creates opportunities for many conversations to happen at the same time. Long introductions and background presentations reduce the opportunity for interaction.

Facilitate Peer-to-Peer Exchange in Large Virtual Events

It's more challenging to promote peer-to-peer learning virtually. For example, there's a trade-off between maximizing the opportunity for discussion by keeping phone lines open and minimizing the possibility of disruption from background noise.

The following are some creative ways to promote peer-to-peer sharing in virtual meetings:

- **On-deck speakers**: If it's not possible to keep lines open for discussion, have two or three participants on an open line who are "on deck" to comment after a presentation about what they heard that was insightful to them and how they could use the information.
- **Polls:** Use polls effectively to engage participants in the dialogue taking place online. For example, if one organization is presenting about an improvement in enrollment, poll the other participants about what percent improvement they think they could achieve by a given date in the near future.
- **Group chat:** Direct participants to group chat immediately after a presentation so they can ask questions of the speaker. Group chats can also provide a mechanism to collect answers to open-ended questions. For example, at the end of a virtual session, let participants enter their action commitments to the group chat. Acknowledge the commitments verbally and within the group chat.

Facilitate Peer-to-Peer Exchange in Small Virtual Events

There are a number of reasons why participants may be reluctant to share their experiences and lessons learned during session activities. The following are some of the challenges that collaborative sponsors may encounter:

- **Lack of rapport in group:** Especially early in the collaborative, it's important to provide opportunities such as in-person learning sessions for participants to build a sense of community and solidarity.
- **Dominant participants:** Sometimes a few participants might dominate a session and it may be difficult to get others to engage. To manage this, consider using the "step up, step back" method for discussion where the moderator occasionally pauses the conversation and acknowledges those who have stepped up to share and then asks them to step back to allow others a chance to contribute.

Create Peer Faculty

One of the key sources of support to participants is from top performing peers who are working toward the same goal. A small group of individuals from these organizations within the collaborative can provide valuable support and coaching to their peers. The faculty becomes part of the larger team that's implementing the learning collaborative and providing guidance on the focus and content of events, feedback on materials, and technical support to their peers, one-to-one or in small groups.

Peer faculty technical support methods include the following:

- **Coaching other participants:** Either one-to-one or in small groups, faculty help their peers share what works for them and what they're learning. They listen to their peers' experiences and action plans, provide them insights and feedback, and coach them on best practices in design, delivery and strategic management of their programs.
- **Reviewing key materials:** Faculty can serve as first reviewers and a sounding board for new materials. The faculty's input is particularly helpful when the materials are complex or introduce new frameworks or concepts.

Encourage faculty to take ownership of and become spokespeople for collaborative materials, indicating that they stand by them at all times.

- **Identifying innovations:** As peers and top performers, faculty have a particularly good ear for innovations. Charge faculty members with the task of listening to the participants that they're coaching for practices that seem particularly innovative or lessons that seem important to spread to others.
- **Spreading activities:** Faculty members are part of the face of the learning collaborative and can be essential spokespeople, internally and externally, for the spread of activities.

Select Faculty Members

Individuals from organizations that are among the most successful in achieving the aims of the collaborative, or at least one particular initiative, should make up the collaborative faculty. The following is useful criteria for selecting peer faculty members:

- **Deep knowledge of their program and factors that have contributed to their success:** Sponsors can help faculty focus on the details of implementation rather than large concepts that may not translate to other settings.
- **Strong commitment to data-driven program management and continuous QI:** When high performers promote an idea, they still have room to improve; this generates more camaraderie and speaks to the core value of striving for excellence.
- **Demonstrated communication and leadership skills:** Peer faculty should be invested in helping others, not simply "bragging" about their successes.

With all of the ways they can contribute to the collaborative, faculty members are investing a fair amount of time. Recognition of peer faculty is necessary, and, if possible, a modest honorarium is helpful for their significant contributions.

Provide Access to Subject-Matter Experts

Subject-matter experts (SMEs) from outside the community can be a valuable complement to peer exchange. SMEs should not be the primary source of ideas for change for the collaborative. That is more common in a traditional learning network. But they can add value in a complementary role to continuous improvement and peer-to-peer exchange.

It's useful to think broadly about what types of expertise will help the collaborative—and about who needs support. Think about the different audiences represented in the collaborative:

- **Leadership:** Wisdom around changes taking place in the delivery system and what the implications are for their organizations; presentations to key audiences like a hospital board or state legislature
- **Managers:** Leadership, QI methods, strategic use of data to drive decision-making
- **Frontline staff:** Clinical, communication, teamwork, leadership, QI

When utilizing SMEs, there are some ways to help get the most out of the relationship:

- **Invest time in prepping them:** SMEs are often most familiar and comfortable in the traditional conference setting. Share background on the work of the collaborative and help them understand the organizations and the community norms so they can make their work relevant to the collaborative. For example, if a part of every event is to engage the participants in a dialogue about what insights they are taking away and how they can apply them to their programs, work with the experts to build that into their presentations to the group. An "interview" format allows for a dialogue between the SME and the audience, when appropriate.

- **Frame their presentations for the collaborative:** If SMEs are presenting to the collaborative, a planning team member should explain why the expert is there, how it's relevant to their work, and what the participants should be thinking about when they're listening to the expert. It's especially important with SMEs to connect the dots for the participants.
- **Consider creative ways for experts to engage with participants:** For example, if they represent a key external stakeholder audience that the collaborative members need to engage with, invite the experts to listen to and provide feedback to members of the collaborative in a coaching capacity.

Build Participant Improvement Capacity and Capability

A critical role of a collaborative sponsor is to assess and, if needed, build the capacity and capability of its members to implement QI methods with discipline and rigor. Understanding the impact of improvements—seeing actual results—makes the exchange of ideas in a collaborative more powerful. Build participants' improvement capacity by helping them monitor their performance, creating feedback loops, and connecting with them at multiple levels of their organizations.

Improve Capacity of Participants to Manage Their Programs with Data

Collaborative sponsors collect data to measure progress toward the aims. Sponsors should establish a norm of reporting the data back to the collaborative regularly.

Data reports should include trends over time showing progress toward goals. When presenting progress toward the aims of the collaborative, structure the data presentations to highlight the following:

- **Top performers:** This is what's possible. Acknowledge and celebrate the top performers. Ask them to talk about what has contributed to their success.
- **Variation in performance across the collaborative:** This is the opportunity. This is why the collaborative exists to help everyone make dramatic breakthroughs in performance, regardless of their starting point, to achieve remarkable results.

Framing data presentations in this way helps the data to serve continuously as a catalyst for action and improvement. If data and resources exist, sponsors should delve deep into the qualitative and quantitative data they collect from participants to identify opportunities for improvement.

Establish a discipline of reviewing available data and perform analyses that may shed light on performance trends. For example, if the sponsor has data on whether the participants implemented a particular practice, the sponsor can look at relevant process measures to see if there's an impact on outcomes.

Sponsors can conduct analyses for participants using their data to show them how they're progressing toward their goals, how their progress compares to that of their peers in the collaborative, what level of performance they'll need to achieve to reach their goals over the duration of the collaborative, and what their priority areas for improvement may be. Over time, the goal is to help participants perform these types of analyses on their own.

Improve Participants' Capacity to Implement QI Methods

Another way sponsors support participants is by helping them build knowledge and skills around QI methods. Participants will come with different skill bases in this area and from organizations with varying levels of commitment to improvement. Sponsors can meet the collaborative participants where they are by assessing their facility with improvement methods and providing targeted levels of support to participants with different needs. For example, some participants may benefit from intensive training—either in person or virtually—to build a foundation in improvement methods. Others might benefit from a brief refresher session. Others with more advanced skills might welcome the opportunity to coach other members of the collaborative.

Whether they come into a collaborative with beginning, intermediate or advanced improvement skills, all would benefit from coaching and feedback from experts in QI. This could take place through one-to-one calls or virtual "office hours" where any participant is invited to call in at a specific time with questions for an expert.

Connect to the Core

Successful collaboratives connect with participating organizations at multiple levels. These organizations should commit to having leaders and staff participate in the collaborative in a meaningful way. This can help the organizations secure the will and the resources necessary to make changes in how they operate. Sponsors can tailor the experience for the three key audiences: leaders, managers and frontline staff.

Connect with Leadership

- Engage leadership early. Support them in leading their organizations toward change. Help them understand the landscape in which the collaborative is taking place—why improvement is necessary and how it will position participating organizations for success.
- Help them understand what resources across their organization will need to be in place for the improvements to occur.
- Help them develop a leadership story they can use internally and externally to build will for making change.

Connect with Implementers

- Implementers are the primary audience of the collaborative. These are the day-to-day leaders within their organizations for implementing changes and improvements.
- Help the implementers strategically manage their work. Provide them support in using improvement methods with discipline and using data effectively.
- Support the implementers in becoming leaders for change. Encourage them to develop their leadership stories (what they stand for) and their leadership voices.
- Help them learn from each other and external experts about what is working. Provide them with successful and actionable strategies from their peers.
- Give them opportunities to interact with each other to learn, share stories and exchange ideas.

Connect with Frontline Staff

- Frontline staff in the participating organizations are those whose work will be most affected by improvements introduced through the collaborative.
- The collaborative may not engage with these staff directly but can provide tools and support to the leadership and implementers to help them become more successful.
- Help leadership and the implementers develop a plan for communicating. Messaging within an organization is crucial for success. Encourage them to highlight their goals in concrete and easy-to-understand terms, seek ideas for improvement from the front line, report back regularly on their progress, and celebrate success.

Create a Culture of Improvement

Creating a culture of improvement is an essential success factor. Collaboratives disrupt what is routine and stimulate participants to action. For the collaborative to succeed, measurement must accompany action. As participants in the collaborative adopt established best practices or promising practices emerging from their peers, it is essential that they measure and track their performance and examine it strategically to understand how they can improve on their results.

Two elements must be in place to establish a culture of QI in a collaborative: an orientation toward outcomes and a strong foundation in QI methods.

Focus on Outcomes

Participants should maintain their focus on achieving the collaborative aims. The collaborative sponsor has a critical role in reinforcing a focus on outcomes by analyzing and reporting performance data, helping participants to understand where they can improve, and coaching participants to improve continuously.

Every interaction with the participants is an opportunity to focus them on outcomes. One of the disciplines to bring to the collaborative is keeping participant presentations brief, focused and data-driven. The most effective presentations are focused on implementation tactics and results. Presentations on participant progress in the collaborative, including the results of implementation, should avoid spending a lot of time on an organization's background, program design and other contextual information.

Collaborative sponsors should prep speakers on effective presentations, including coaching them on using their data to tell a story and keeping their presentations focused on the change they tested and outcomes it produced. It may be helpful to have a presentation template, or models of effective presentations, and to provide limits on time and the number of slides allowed.

Understand QI Methods

An effective collaborative marries an outcomes orientation with skill building in QI methods. QI is an ongoing, participatory process. Even well-validated QI strategies require adaptation to local needs and the skills to address both technical and cultural aspects of change. Training in QI will accelerate participants' abilities to create an environment for change. They will learn and apply the principles and tools of improvement science, better equipping them to elaborate, refine and execute on their efforts to make improvements.

Hands-on, project-based learning is the best way to gain a firm grounding in the concepts, tools and methods needed for an effective QI journey.

When providing support in QI methods, a few key considerations are germane:

- **Skill sets:** Sponsors should recognize that the participants will come in with different levels of skill. Some will need basic training in QI methods, designing and implementing PDSAs, and measuring their performance with data. Others may have a solid foundation in QI methods but would benefit from coaching and feedback. Sponsors can meet participants where they are by adopting flexible and different modes of QI support (e.g., a mix of didactic sessions, office hours and feedback on participants' QI activities).

- **Commitment to QI:** Another aspect of meeting participants where they are is recognizing that participants are part of larger organizations and the QI culture will vary across their organizations. Some participants may encounter more challenges in gaining institutional support for implementing tests of change and accessing the data and organizational resources they need. These participants might need extra support and dedicated time to share their lessons learned with participants in a similar situation.

- **Learning from experts and each other:** The richest learning will take place if the participants have opportunities to learn from experts in QI and to learn from each other. From improvement experts, they gain a solid foundation in improvement methods. They also benefit from feedback on their QI plans, including designing, implementing and measuring the success and interpreting their findings. Learning from each other, they also gain insights and practical strategies.

- **Training and feedback:** Much of the focus of a collaborative is on peer-to-peer exchange of insights and learnings. It can be beneficial to provide a foundation in QI methods through a more didactic training approach.

A more traditional training program can take place in-person or virtually, be time limited, and doesn't need to span the duration of the collaborative. It's probably more helpful to concentrate these trainings early in the collaborative to develop core improvement skills. Following the training, provide coaching to participants, either in one-to-one or small group sessions to reinforce their skills.

Be in Improvement Mode

Another way that a sponsor can create a culture of improvement is by modeling it in the implementation of the collaborative. Sponsors can model the discipline of testing changes and being in continuous improvement by:

- **Being transparent:** If you're trying out a new format for a session, tell participants this and ask for their feedback.
- **Adapting based on data:** Adapt quickly to participant feedback. If running a multi-day learning session, make time each day to review feedback and make any changes to the plans for the following day. Start the next day with a report on the feedback and how you're addressing it.

Participants achieve a culture of improvement in the collaborative when they view QI methods as an integral part of how they approach their work rather than as a project they do in addition to their work.

Conclusion

The collaborative model can be a powerful engine for breakthrough improvements in how healthcare is delivered. Sponsors of collaboratives can position themselves for success by optimizing the effectiveness of the participants. They can do this by creating a sense of urgency to achieve a shared goal, building a community with open exchange of ideas, providing technical assistance and support to participants, and creating a culture of improvement.

[1] Wenger, E. (1998). Communities of practice: learning as a social system. *The Systems Thinker* , 9 (5).

[2] Bisognano, M. (2013, Apr.). All Teach, All Learn. *International Forum on Quality and Safety in Healthcare* , Speech.

CHAPTER 9

Flexible Design and Funding of Large-Scale Collaboratives

By Stephen Hines, Ph.D. and James B. Battles, Ph.D.
Resourcing, Marketing and Self-Funding a
Collaborative by Andrea Kabcenell, RN, MPH
Investing in Patient Safety and Quality by Marybeth Sharpe, Ph.D.

Introduction

Healthcare lacks a coordinated infrastructure for the diffusion, implementation and adoption of evidence-based safe practices to improve the quality and safety of healthcare. A patient safety practice has been defined as a type of process or structure whose application reduces the probability of adverse events resulting from exposure to the healthcare system across the range of diseases and procedures.[1] While evidence of best practices exists, translating that evidence into practice and getting it adopted represents a significant problem.[2] For organizations wishing to make improvements in healthcare, major considerations include selecting which safe practices or innovations to diffuse and how to carry out the diffusion or adoption of activities at the target scale: local, regional or national.

A funding agency must make several important decisions before launching any large-scale improvement project, including 1) what's to be improved, 2) what's the safe practice leading to the desired improvement, and 3) how to get frontline providers to adopt the safe practice. If there's no safe practice that exists for the desired improvement, the effort isn't ready for large-scale diffusion activities,

and the project is really a process to help develop safe practices, not implementation or adoption. This chapter focuses on the components of designing and funding large-scale collaboratives.

Design Parameters

Funders of large-scale collaboratives should carefully consider two major design parameters. First, selecting the campaign's topic or focus is essential. Second, choosing the length of the initiative is equally critical to ensure it uses resources effectively.

Topic Selection

Funders of large-scale projects must make choices regarding where they'll invest in improving the healthcare system. Following are some questions to guide these decisions.

First, is there clear evidence of a gap between current practice and what constitutes optimal quality, safety, equitability, efficiency or whatever aim the collaborative is targeting? Without clear evidence of a gap, it will be difficult to show substantial improvement and even recruit providers to participate in the campaign. While seemingly obvious, there have been collaboratives where baseline rates of harm were so low that any additional improvement was very difficult to achieve. On the other hand, Institute for Healthcare Improvement's 100,000 Lives Campaign and the recently completed Hospital Engagement Network (HEN) funded by Centers for Medicare & Medicaid Services (CMS) are good examples of collaboratives that did a good job presenting compelling data that substantial improvement was possible.

A second question to ask is whether tools and process changes are known to significantly reduce the gap between the current and optimal practices. While collaborative leaders may need to assemble and organize resources to support the project, there should be clear evidence that the resources exist and can lead to substantial improvements in a diverse range of settings.

Many improvements developed within a single healthcare setting may work, but may depend on unique characteristics of the particular setting that don't exist in other locations. Systemwide or regional proofs of concept that demonstrate how a particular approach is scalable should normally exist before a funder invests in a large-scale campaign. For example, the Agency for Healthcare Research and Quality (AHRQ)-funded Comprehensive Unit-Based Safety Program (CUSP) at the national level utilized practice changes learned from the Keystone initiative in the state of Michigan reduced central-line-associated bloodstream infection (CLABSI).

The third question funders should ask regarding the topics they choose to invest in is whether the timing is appropriate. Investing in collaboratives too soon can result in substantial waste if it can't get traction with key stakeholders, is not made a priority by providers it seeks to target, and lacks compelling evidence that substantial improvement is possible. If this is the case, funders could reduce their risk by investing in smaller local or regional collaborative efforts that may help create the evidence needed for a successful national campaign. Another scenario is investing in large-scale campaigns focused on topics that are already being successfully improved upon and competing with these efforts. Instead, funders might use their resources to enhance the impact of the existing efforts.

Project Time Span

After topic selection, choosing an appropriate duration for a national collaborative is a second key design parameter. Funders sometimes must define the lengths of initiatives based on factors outside their control. But to whatever extent possible, their decisions about how long collaboratives should be funded should be guided by several key considerations.

Availability of Raw Materials: When improvement resources already exist, large-scale collaboratives obviously require less time than those lacking the raw materials. But even when tools pre-exist, national collaboratives also require leadership teams that include multiple content experts and a viable infrastructure capable of supporting the collaborative at the local or regional levels. At least six months is required to fully organize and equip the national and local supporters so they can support participant improvement efforts. If tools must be developed and campaign staff must be trained to use them, it will probably require a year for this phase.

Implementation Complexity: Some innovations that improve care can be implemented quite quickly, while others are far more complex. Funders should talk with those who have successfully implemented innovations to understand how long their efforts took.

While it may be tempting to assume that making improvements during the collaborative will take less time than implementing innovations because tools and process changes already exist, in fact, innovators tend to make changes more rapidly than many of their peers. When estimating project duration, funders should include the time required to 1) convince facilities to make the improvement a priority (the recruitment period), 2) implement recommended changes (the intervention period), and 3) embed these changes into the organizational culture and normal work patterns (the sustainability phase). Times required for each of these activities will vary greatly depending on the topic. In general, when the improvement case is compelling, recruitment is faster.

Changes that require relatively simple actions by a small number of people take far less time than changes that require many people to make

Investing in Patient Safety and Quality

By Marybeth Sharpe, Ph.D.

Funders have options for investing their philanthropic dollars toward improving patient safety and quality. They may directly support providers' quality improvement activities, invest in research or seed new technologies, to name a few. The Gordon and Betty Moore Foundation chose among these and other options by launching several San Francisco Bay Area collaboratives.

The Moore Foundation made this investment to multiply and accelerate the improvement efforts of individual hospitals. With a focus on pragmatic learning, hospitals shared the specifics of how they implemented evidence-based practices at the bedside. Collaboratives also enabled engagement of frontline clinicians, particularly registered nurses, in peer-to-peer learning and regional leadership.

Funding a collaborative involves matching budget to its goals, the improvement capacity of its participants, the external environment and the topics addressed. For a collaborative with specific quantitative improvement goals, the Moore Foundation built in funding for technical assistance, clinical experts and in-person meetings. Technical assistance by clinicians was instrumental to achieving improvement goals across all Bay Area hospitals, an explicit aspiration of this particular collaborative. In the case of a learning network with less specific goals and a more targeted group of participants, the Moore Foundation budgeted less technical assistance and clinician

many changes in a coordinated way. For example, dramatic reductions in the number of early elective deliveries occurred quite rapidly—probably because the changes only required the decision by a person or small set of people to change organizational policies and did not require technical or clinical changes. On the other hand, national catheter-associated urinary tract infection (CAUTI) rates have declined slowly and moderately—probably because it requires changes to entrenched practices by many clinicians.

While funders don't need to be clinical experts, they should understand the complexity of the changes required before they set the length of collaboratives that they choose to fund. Failure to budget sufficient time for all of these phases is likely to have three outcomes funders will regret: inadequate recruitment, promotion of easy solutions over more difficult yet impactful ones, and poor sustainability.

Data Lag: As health information technology systems become more widespread, the time between when patient harms occur and when data is available documenting those harms has declined. While we expect this desirable trend to continue, funders still should carefully consider the impact of data lag on the duration of projects they fund. For example, due to data lag issues in the past, Quality Improvement Organizations (QIOs) sometimes had readmission re-measurement periods that ended before many of their readmission reduction activities had even begun. Another example is when final reports that summarize the impact of the project are due at the same time the intervention period ends. When possible, no-cost extensions may give projects sufficient time to analyze data when a project ends. Alternatively, building in the time required for data collection and analysis will prevent either the premature end of needed improvement activities or the failure to capture the full impact of a project due to incomplete data.

Limited Attention Span: A final consideration for funders in determining the length of collaboratives relates to the attention span of project participants. Active engagement in collaboratives rarely extends more than a year, except on very complex topics; and six months is more common. While sustainability and monitoring activities may continue (as well as work on other topics, as was common in the HEN initiative), campaign designs that assume active interventions for longer periods should be carefully examined to ensure that project participants view this extra time as desirable. Providers face a rapidly changing environment with many opportunities for improvements. Funders should recognize the limited attention spans of providers and ensure their collaborative durations reflect this inevitability.

Funding Mechanisms and Budget Flexibility: Federal agencies and private non-government organizations (NGO) such as foundations can fund large-scale improvement projects or they can be self-funded by participating organizations. An example of self-funding of smaller collaboratives designed around specific topics is highlighted in a case study from the IHI.

time. External environment is also a consideration, as regulatory incentives for improvement may enable match funding from participants. And a collaborative addressing an emerging issue may require more funding than a collaborative addressing a topic with existing attention and resources.

These considerations can help funders and collaborative leaders align on a budget that achieves their common goals for improving patient care.

Case Study: Resourcing, Marketing and Self-Funding a Collaborative

By Andrea Kabcenell, RN, MPH

An Institute for Healthcare Improvement (IHI) Breakthrough Series (BTS) collaborative is an example of a self-funded collaborative.[3] It brings together a group of organizations to achieve a specific aim during a specified time period, alternating between learning sessions, in which teams learn and plan tests of change, and action periods, in which teams test changes in their organizations, receive coaching and report back on results. BTS collaboratives are designed to help from 30 to 130 teams achieve breakthrough results, such as 50 percent reduction in hospital mortality or emergency wait times.

Because collaboratives use an "all teach, all learn" approach, the number of teams determines only the room size and catering, not the staffing. Collaboratives typically last six to 15 months; those with more complex changes or within complicated systems take more time. Table 1 shows the resources considered essential for teaching, collaborating and coaching.

Personnel	Days per Month Required
Director	4-6
Project manager and coordinator	7
Meeting planner	1
Improvement advisor	1.5-3
Expert faculty (one to three people)	3-4
Other resources Meeting space, faculty travel, marketing and communications	

Table 1. Sample costs associated with Breakthrough Series Collaborative

To market a collaborative, IHI sends out an email call for applications and publicizes the collaborative's aims at meetings and with lists of likely participants. Most IHI programs are funded by user fees. Organizations that pay their own way are highly motivated and engaged, and they usually have the strong leadership support that drives success.

The fees are paid by individual organizations or by large corporate bodies—government grants or corporate offices. At times, foundations or others will pay for or supplement tuition to allow safety-net organizations or others to participate. To assure breaking even on collaboratives, IHI regularly uses attraction strategies such as identifying and publicizing the most likely positive return on investment for the participants and creating incentives for enrollment like group discounts for large healthcare systems. To balance revenue and expense, the IHI calculates a break-even number of teams and market accordingly while building flexibility in faculty contracts to use less or more of their time as needed.

The type of organization sponsoring the effort also may influence the type of mechanisms that can be used to fund such activities. There are two basic types of funding mechanisms: grants and contracts.

Grants are a form of gift from the funding organizations to the receiving organization to carry out the desired work. The grant allows a good deal of freedom to the receiving organization in the execution of the project. Contracts are basically work-for-hire, with the funding organization directing the nature of the project, with a defined scope of work and a set time schedule and specified deliverables as part of the contract.

Federal agencies more often use grants for developmental work and contracts for specific implantation or diffusion activities. With grants, the receiving organization is responsible to the management of execution of the project with minimal direction from the funding organization. The relationship between funding and receiving organizations is reversed when a contract is used. The funding organization directs the scope of work and provides a good deal more oversight and control of the work for hire. Contract mechanisms are favored by most federal agencies for large-scale projects because of budgetary size.

Federal contracting is a very tightly controlled process dictated by a complex set of regulations as outlined in Federal Acquisition Regulation (FAR) rules. The FAR dictates who can bid on contract proposals and the nature of the final contract and payment approach, such as fixed price or cost reimbursement plus fee. Solicitation for contracts can be full and open competition or can be limited competition for funding.

Fixed-price contracts are an advantage for the funding organization because the total cost of the project is determined in advance and the contractor must deliver the specified work at the price agreed upon. If the work costs more than the estimate, the contractor must absorb those costs. However, if the work actually costs less, the contractor is paid the full amount. Fixed-price contracts are best used when the work is well-defined and is not subject to uncontrolled variables that are not under the control of the funding agency or the contractor.

Cost reimbursement contracts pose fewer risks to the contractor because the direct costs of the work are reimbursed, plus a fee is paid to cover the margin. Usually the fee is fixed. A cost reimbursement contract can be advantageous to a funding agency when the possibility of unanticipated costs or outside variables could increase the costs. The cost reimbursement contract provides slightly more flexibility for both funder and contractor.

Funders should recognize that despite the good intentions of the organizations with whom they work, the structure of project funding may affect how projects are staffed and executed. Funders should anticipate how the payment approach they are using may affect the execution of the project and discuss their expectations with the organizations they fund. For example, CMS required at least some prospective HEN contractors to provide written assurances that any unspent resources from their fixed-price contracts would be spent to advance the goals of its Partnership for Patients initiative.

When funders require funds budgeted for specific project years to be spent in those years, they should carefully review budgets to ensure they reflect varying expenditure patterns. Startup costs often depend on whether an existing infrastructure is in place, such as with ongoing communities and networks, or whether hiring, recruitment and other ramp-up costs are necessary. Likewise, ongoing networks may finish "at full steam," anticipating a new project will start immediately at the conclusion of another. While new individual projects or national campaigns have different start-up and wind-down periods and activities than continual networks, funders should consider adjusting the timing of budgeting and expenditures based on different funding needs.

Funders should also ensure that funding mechanisms allow the flexibility to shift resources between budget categories relatively easily. It's highly unlikely that budgets for large-scale, multi-year collaboratives can anticipate exactly how resources will need to be allocated. Significant change is predictable during large-scale improvement efforts. Funders should anticipate and support these changes by ensuring they can quickly adjust contracts and budgets to support the project's needs.

Project Management

Funders vary greatly with respect to the approaches they use to oversee the progress of national collaboratives. A preferred strategy is the one recommended for the governing boards of organizations: providing defined goals, defining clear processes for overseeing progress toward these goals, and ensuring there is agreement about how progress toward defined goals will be evaluated.

Project Goals

When organizations receive grants or contracts from funders, they want to meet or exceed their expectations, but sometimes the overarching goals for projects are fuzzily defined and the funding organization's goals for a project differ from the goals of the organization's project officer. Well-defined goals contribute significantly to success. Without them, large-scale collaboratives commonly fail. While goals may vary, the following are some recommendations:

- Funders should ensure that they have one or more clearly defined goals for collaboratives before they commit to funding them, such as CMS's HEN initiative (40 percent reduction in specific harm measures, 20 percent reduction in readmissions), IHI's 100,000 Lives Campaign and

AHRQ's CUSP-CLABSI initiative. These goals were clear and reflected an awareness of current levels of performance as well as the amount they felt the campaigns could improve those levels. Even when the primary goal is clear, funders often have secondary goals that they should articulate and share with the organizations they choose to lead these efforts. Philanthropies may want the collaborative to raise their visibility; federal agencies may want their projects to facilitate enhanced coordination with other federal partners. Reducing disparities may be as important to the funder as improving overall rates. In all these cases, it is easier to define and execute a strategy when the goals are clearly shared with those providing operational leadership for the initiative.

- Funders should have a substantive discussion of their primary and secondary goals during a collaborative's kick-off meeting and at regular intervals thereafter. Conversations about these goals in which secondary goals are identified, tensions between goals are discussed, and priorities are clarified are extremely valuable. This is particularly true on projects where considerable time passes between when a funder decides to fund a large-scale collaborative and when it actually commences.

- Funders should make changes to goals when they are needed. There have been multiple collaboratives in which initial goals proved unachievable, or they achieved the goals so rapidly that they became irrelevant. AHRQ recently funded an initiative with a primary goal to reduce surgical site infections in ambulatory surgical centers. But the emergence of data suggesting that the rates of these infections were very low and the recognition that most procedures performed in ambulatory surgery centers don't involve incisions (making surgical site infections impossible) led AHRQ to conclude it should expand the initial goals to encompass a broader range of potential harms.

Project Oversight and Timelines

Funders typically require proposals for large-scale collaboratives to include detailed plans for project implementation and timelines reflecting when specific activities will occur. Quite often these activities are written into the contract, and sometimes milestones in the delivery schedule are even linked to project payments. While aligning goals with contractual requirements and with payment is good practice, large-scale collaboratives require a different approach to project planning and timelines than an approach that works well for many research and resource development projects. Following are key recommendations to funders that capture the most important of these differences.

First, funders should only link the broadest and most important milestones and objectives to contracting requirements and payments. Because changes are predictable, linking too many details to the contract risks substantial inefficiencies associated with multiple contract modifications. But an even greater risk is that the collaborative will persist with approaches the team believes are inferior simply because they're in the contractual requirements.

Second, planning documents should adjust and adapt based on experience and progress. It's a maxim in war that "no battle plan ever survives contact with the enemy." This logic also applies to plans for large-scale collaboratives. Initial efforts to recruit participants and support their improvement efforts inevitably surface both opportunities for improvements and challenges that must be addressed. Moreover, as the collaborative proceeds, some challenges recede and new ones replace them. At the start of the AHRQ-funded CUSP-CLABSI project, the team spent considerable time convincing hospitals that CLABSI was a significant problem and that the recommended changes were capable of significantly reducing it. Several years later, published evidence had become widely accepted and a new challenge emerged: convincing hospitals that they could not easily fix their CLABSI problems without external assistance.

Because substantial changes are predictable, and predicting what those changes will be is not, initial project-planning documents work best if they reflect high-level plans for executing all the dimensions of the entire collaborative but only provide details for the initial six months of the project.

Third, funders should require regular reviews and updates to the collaborative's overall strategy and project plan. Such an approach acknowledges the need for ongoing updates to strategy and tactics and avoids the risk of executing outdated plans. National collaboratives pose substantial communication challenges. Providing too much long-range detail almost inevitably creates a need to announce more changes to these details, which can lead to both confusion and a belief that that collaborative is being poorly led. An incremental approach to project planning holds off on finalizing details and announcing them to project participants until decisions about tactics must be made. This allows the project leadership to articulate a clear overall strategy and acknowledge that future activities will be finalized based on what happens in earlier phases of the collaborative and creates an expectation that change is normal and good, versus an expectation that change is a response to planning errors and failures.

Fourth, funders should review project plans to ensure that strategies and tactics evolve over the course of the collaborative. Successful national collaboratives should observe two important changes that will require them to use different approaches in later phases than they did at the outset of the campaign. First, effective campaigns should change the external environment. They should create greater awareness of the targeted problem, lessen skepticism that the problem can be reduced, and create awareness of tools and approaches that will support collaborative efforts.

Finally, project plans should address the change in the prototypical project participant. Engaging with innovators and early adopters is very different from supporting late majority or laggard project participants. While a multi-cohort project may include participants at many points on the diffusion-of-innovation curve, plans that assume later cohorts will have the same needs and orientation to change as the counterparts from the earlier cohorts are probably quite flawed. The groups are usually quite different and will require different types and levels of support. Strategies for leveraging participants from earlier cohorts to support later ones are particularly valuable because later cohorts will find recommendations from their peers more compelling than ones from national experts.

Project Evaluation

Evaluating the impact of their programs is a prime objective of most funders. While funders may not possess the expertise to create evaluation plans for large-scale collaboratives, they can define expectations related to project evaluation that are likely to maximize the impact of their investments. Following are some recommendations.

Changes in Processes and Outcomes: Funders should ensure that the evaluation encompasses both changes in processes and changes in outcomes. Though process changes may not inevitably translate into improved outcomes, some processes such as recruitment and data submission are absolutely essential to provable changes in outcomes. Moreover, because these and other processes will precede changes in outcomes, they're often leading indicators in the earlier phases of a project. Without data that shows that collaborative participants made changes to their culture or clinical practices, improved outcomes may be attributed to secular trends or other factors totally disconnected to the collaborative. All of these factors make it important to ensure that the evaluation design captures the changes in key processes.

Evaluating outcomes is equally important. Standards of evidence required to prove that campaigns have achieved their goals are steadily increasing. Even when reported outcomes improve from a baseline to a defined re-measurement period some design choices can make it difficult to provide evidence that the project was a demonstrably good investment. These include: the failure to ensure the baseline closely precedes the time period for improvement activities, a failure to establish some level of data integrity, and the inability to demonstrate greater levels of outcome improvement among project participants than among nonparticipants.

Reliable, Feasible and Timely Measures: Ensure that all chosen process and outcome measures are reasonably reliable, feasible and timely. The burden of data collection poses a major obstacle to the recruitment and retention of collaborative participants. Using existing, validated or endorsed measures (as well as standardized methods for collecting and reporting them) represents a good evaluation strategy. Moreover, using measures that participants may already collect and report to CMS or CDC can reduce data burden. Funders should also insure that any measures they view as critical to the evaluation can be collected in a reasonably timely way. Measures based on claims data usually suffer from substantial data lag and should be avoided if other more timely options exist.

Stated Goals: Ensure that all project goals are captured in the project evaluation. Expanded recruitment efforts are likely to attract participants that may be less committed or capable of producing substantial improvements in outcomes. And depending on how goals are defined, recruiting facilities with very good rates at the outset of the project may be a very good strategy, if the stated goal is based on the overall rate at the end of the project—or a very bad strategy, if the stated goal is based on the amount of observed improvement from project start to end. In addition to the number of participants, funders should consider whether they want to evaluate them so that they can understand if recruitment efforts failed to attract low performers or facilities serving disadvantaged populations.

Formative and Summative Evaluation Activities: Funders should require both formative and summative evaluation activities for large-scale spread efforts they support. Formative evaluation activities serve two important roles.

First, they provide the funder with data on progress that it can use to ensure its investments are on a desirable trajectory. Second, and more importantly, the data provides the project leaders with information they should be using to make mid-course adjustments to strengthen the impact of the campaign. Any large-scale collaborative that lacks the collection and ongoing use of data to guide planning is lacking an essential element and probably should not be funded before adjustments are made.

Summative evaluations offer the best, retrospective evidence about how well a collaborative met stated goals. While evaluation plans may evolve as a collaborative progresses, a plausible plan for conducting the summative evaluation must exist from the start of the project to ensure that the data it requires will be available when the project ends. Sometimes funders hire an external evaluator to conduct this evaluation. While this approach can yield results that are more credible, it still requires that the evaluation plan is developed early on and that there is effective coordination between the evaluator and the project lead to ensure that needed data is available.

Perspective and Priorities: Funders should ensure that evaluation activities remain secondary to the primary goal of achieving large-scale improvements in the healthcare system. Project teams or funders that include strong evaluators who seek to contribute to the pool of generalizable knowledge may prioritize the data collection activities to a level that seriously compromises the ability to recruit project participants. If the research and evaluation activities become the primary focus, the large-scale collaborative will probably morph into a much smaller-scale research project with much cleaner data obtained from fewer representative participants and appreciably less spread and impact on patients.

Conclusion

Designing and funding large-scale collaboratives for the diffusion and adoption of safe practices is challenging for both the funding agency that chooses to fund such activities as well as the organizations willing to accept the responsibility to carry out such projects. These are field-based-type projects that must bring value to the healthcare organizations that are to adopt the innovations or safe practices. While challenging, these types of projects are particularly rewarding in their ability to provide the technical assistance necessary for healthcare organizations to adopt safe practices to improve the quality and safety of care they provide.

---

[1] Shekelle, P., Wachter, R., Pronovost, P., Schoelles, K., McDonald, K., Dy, S., et al. (2013, March). Making Health Care Safer II: An Updated Critical Analysis of the Evidence for Patient Safety Practices. Comparative Effectiveness Review.

[2] Shekelle, P., Wachter, R., Pronovost, P., Schoelles, K., McDonald, K., Dy, S., et al. (2013, March). Making Health Care Safer II: An Updated Critical Analysis of the Evidence for Patient Safety Practices. *Comparative Effectiveness Review*.

[3] The Breakthrough Series: IHI's Collaborative Model for Achieving Breakthrough Improvement. (2003). *IHI Innovation Series white paper.* Boston: Institute for Healthcare Improvement.

CHAPTER 10

Translating Knowledge into Action

By Karen Wolk Feinstein, Ph.D. and Bruce Block, M.D.
Lean Daily Management Generates Action by John B. Chessare, M.D., MPH

Case study: Lean Daily Management Generates Action

By John B. Chessare, M.D., MPH

In the spring of 2013, leaders at GBMC HealthCare, which owns Greater Baltimore Medical Center, were concerned that the corporation was improving its performance at too slow a pace. The senior executive team was looking for a way to create an organization of focused problem-solvers, and as a result it decided to implement the technique called "lean daily management" (LDM).

LDM is a system that fosters a daily structured interchange between frontline managers and their people and senior leaders of the organization about its four aims: the best possible health outcomes, the best possible care experience, with the least waste and the most joy for those providing the care.

Each unit or department manager oversees the development of one opportunity for improvement and a declared goal under each of the four aims. On a daily basis, including weekends and holidays, the unit or department presents to senior leaders its results from the previous calendar day on elements it's working to improve. The senior leaders thank the teams for their work, stimulate tests of change and remove barriers to improvement that are beyond the ability of the team to remove. Additionally, every morning, before their unit rounds, the senior leaders gather in the executive office and review their own LDM metrics. They then break into five sub-teams to visit the units. The morning meeting and subsequent rounds represent a one- to two-hour daily commitment for all senior leaders.

As a result of using this structured process, issues are identified and solutions are found. As an example, the Post-Anesthesia Care Unit identified that it was not always completing the post-anesthesia evaluation before discharging post-operative patients from the unit. While there hadn't been any significant major events with people leaving who weren't stable, some near misses had occurred, and the team was concerned about potential negative health outcomes. It began to report the daily number of discharges, the number who had left without the form being completed and signed by the anesthesiologist, and the reason why the form hadn't been completed.

The team then tested changes and ultimately created a new process that resulted in 100 percent compliance over many days. The new process became standard work and was documented on a visual display that was available for review at any time by staff members. This metric was ultimately replaced by a new metric under the aim of better health.

LDM is an effective tool because it aligns all units with the overall aims of the organization and engages the workforce in daily tests of change to meet theses aims. It's action-oriented, utilizes the plan-do-study-act (PDSA) cycle to generate improvement, and encourages spread of meaningful change from one unit or department to the next.

Committing to the use of a system such as LDM has enabled Greater Baltimore Medical Center to clearly focus on its aims and persistently pursue them to produce dramatically improved outcomes. It has made many significant improvements under all four aims (best possible health outcomes, best possible care experience, less waste and most joy for providers) since implementing LDM, including the following examples:

- Lowest severity adjusted readmission rates in the state
- Skin breakdowns reduced to zero
- Major improvements in patient engagement scores
- Employee injuries reduced by more than 50 percent

Introduction

Many assume that action follows knowledge. But information provided at conferences and meetings must compete with other sources of knowledge: revealed insight, expert advice, distilled experience, biased perceptions and hunches. Even when learners accept new knowledge, many factors affect the resulting action. Because knowledge doesn't always, or even perhaps often, result in the desired action, this chapter explores how to control the direction and efficacy of action, not just through enhancing the impact of knowledge but also through connecting that knowledge to other precursors of action.

Context of Behavior Change

Learners who can't connect new information to an active concern are less likely to use that knowledge to inform action. A good example of this is relying on the weight of facts to stimulate action—handing brochures to patients and journal articles to providers only to be disappointed when behavior doesn't change or changes very slowly.

Needs, Desires, Aspirations

It's no surprise that simply creating a guideline, protocol or even order sets doesn't generate significant adoption. A better approach is attaching the desired outcome to achievement of personal goals. For example, when working with a physician's office, the initial question is not, "Did you use the guideline?" but rather, "Have you been able to improve the number of call-backs from your asthma patients?" Linking knowledge to tangible, concrete and meaningful results that collaborative participants aspire to helps create a tight bond and promote adoption.

Feelings, Beliefs and Values

Thoughtful, professional education usually de-emphasizes sharing personal beliefs. Unfortunately, this means that professionals don't encourage patients and families to share their own beliefs. Trainers and coaches working with healthcare professionals who drive change in their organizations find many often have strong beliefs that can't be ignored because they are a vehicle, and a potential barrier, for translating knowledge into action. And credible trainers who are good at facilitation and gain acceptance of collaboratives often have to minimize their own biases and opinions. Facilitators have to be open to ideas that contradict their own, to welcome new perspectives to augment their own, and to accept the worthiness of group members who think differently.

Knowledge and Experience

The way knowledge is shared also makes an impact on adoption and subsequent action. Push-back commonly follows beliefs such as, "We're already providing very good care to our patients." In the past, these self-assessments of quality were based on selective memory because the data was often delayed, inaccurate or not specific to the team, provider or organization involved. Now that more current, even real-time, data is available and accurate, providers can see numbers in a more meaningful way.

Knowledge of care deficits may motivate some providers or organizations to seek solutions. However, when providers believe they are already working as hard as they can and are dealing with regulatory and reimbursement pressures and rapid changes in the healthcare system, such knowledge may induce defensiveness, which often obstructs meaningful action. It's usually better to build remedial interventions upon positive goals and accomplishments of an organization rather than upon menacing consequences and judgments.

Experts may lose influence by presenting knowledge as dogma. Creating a sense of joint discovery in the application of facts, data and adaptation enhances adoption. Otherwise, participants may not identify with the expert, may believe the expert doesn't understand the local challenges, or may dismiss a practice as "something that won't work here." A common strategy to overcome this reluctance is to ask participants, even frontline staff, "How would we have to adapt this practice to make it work here?" Acknowledge local issues and the need to generate local ownership of the solution.

Collaboratives in Different Flavors

Behavior change takes place in practices, hospitals and skilled nursing units but can't proceed without the creation of internal champions and change agents.

The "knowledge expert" trainer or facilitator can help build a vision of a more ideal state and help create enthusiasm for and a belief in that vision. But the ultimate purpose of any collaborative is to create internal champions embedded in their organizations, to advance the vision through continuous quality improvements and to ultimately sustain momentum. This is true whether the collaborative uses small or large problem-solving or location-specific groups; a conference format; a one-time special event or training; special quality improvement fellowships; or champion programs.

Above all, the best experiences create a sense of joint discovery and ownership of the vision or goal; confidence that each participant can advance the goal in some way; "mental maps" of significant areas of focus; and small wins that build confidence that improvements are attainable.

Importance of the Messenger

Knowledge adoption and action are also influenced by the context in which information is received. A key factor is the person or persons sharing the information. Because healthcare is a local phenomenon and the context of various participants may vary dramatically, it's important to find "messengers" who can approximate the situation of the different participants. The quintessential role for "peer-to-peer" learning so prominent in most collaboratives builds on this very concept.

The most relevant expert to someone whom we hope to influence and translate knowledge into action is often someone who "looks like them," in terms of the work they do in a similar setting. An academic practice or medical center is more likely to "hear" another person from that setting. A rural hospital nurse is more likely to integrate knowledge from a similarly placed colleague. This also works for senior leaders where a CEO may listen to another leader but is more likely to be activated when a CEO from a similar type of organization shares how it works for them. Peers make knowledge more accessible than many experts, simply because they prove it can work in context-specific situations. The knowledge, and its impact, has already generalized beyond the subject-matter expert into other environments.

Readiness, Support and Activation

The alignment of goals, engagement of values and sharing of knowledge are important determinants of behavior, but the organization and its staff must be ready to change. Dr. James Prochaska's transtheoretical model of behavior change,[1] also known as the "stages of change," which assesses an individual's readiness to act on a new behavior and provides a process for change, can also be applied to organizations. Successful change results from an understanding of motivations for change, awareness of deficits and gaps, prior history of efforts to improve quality, and organizational reserve to understand where best to start working on small "wins."

Collaborative participants arrive in varying stages of readiness and willingness to implement improvements. This situation requires building personal belief in the change upfront and then considering how to build organizational will to eventually attain wholesale adoption and implementation. A powerful way to build will is to use storytelling by a comparable peer about how an innovation or new practice was adopted and the impact it had. This is the essence of the "viral spread" of information and the building of a community of shared interest and knowledge.

Opportunity and Building of Organizational Will

Healthcare providers often feel stuck in a system that cannot administer to the needs of their patients or their workforce. They may feel unable to give excellent care or achieve excellent outcomes. They frequently feel overwhelmed, especially by meaningless and burdensome new tasks and responsibilities. Lack of opportunity deadens their efforts. It's then necessary to help clinicians revisit their original professional aspirations and project them into a future without limits: "What would your practice/unit look like if you could build it the way it should be?" Returning to this vision reinvigorates efforts to overcome obstacles. Opportunity reawakens motivation.

Even with motivated clinicians, without alignment among frontline staff, middle management and senior leaders, improvement activities they promote may not get traction or be prioritized by the organization as a whole. Building organizational will is a frequent duty for participants and collaborative leaders to translate knowledge into action.

Elimination of Hospital Infections

In 1994, Harvard School of Public Health professor Lucian Leape, M.D., warned that "... 180,000 people die each year partly as a result of iatrogenic injury, the equivalent of three jumbo-jet crashes every two days."[2]

Leape's observation motivated a small team of non-clinical professionals working with the Jewish Healthcare Foundation to call for observations in local hospital intensive care units. They found error-prone environments where problems rarely received root-cause interventions, while staff engaged in ever-increasing workarounds. Role confusion, poor handoffs, unreliable support systems and unproven care rituals attested to the absence of quality improvement methods.[3] This report energized the health foundation staff to seek systems-based solutions that had worked in industry to address expensive and harmful errors in healthcare.

First, the foundation approached the business community to authorize a "working together consortium" of health leadership to address these problems. The objective was to make the Pittsburgh region a beacon for the nation. Then it turned to Paul O'Neill, the CEO who had made Alcoa the safest corporation in the world, to help it address medical errors and co-chair the consortium, along with Karen Feinstein, CEO of Jewish Healthcare Foundation (JHF). With support from regional CEOs, the consortium came to be called Pittsburgh Regional Health Initiative (PRHI). O'Neill invited the JHF team and sympathetic health professionals to attend Alcoa University, where they learned the fundamentals of the Toyota Production System (TPS), a popular lean method of quality improvement.

Gathered in the large Alcoa conference room were more than 50 leaders of local health systems, hospitals and practices representing management, medicine, nursing and pharmacy. They came partly out of curiosity but brought with them a great deal of skepticism. One participant said, "Those people at PRHI are talking about perfect outcomes! What do they know about clinical care and challenges of unpredictable and largely unavoidable complications? Hospital care can't be run like a factory."

Competing healthcare providers and payers continued to come to meetings because of O'Neill's stature and the stewardship of the business community—no one could afford to let others gain an advantage in claiming dedication to quality.

Leadership from more than 30 regional hospitals reached consensus: They would work together with Centers for Disease Control and Prevention to tackle central line–associated bloodstream infections (CLABs). The idea was to focus on just one problem and carefully measure the results. All members of the care team were activated. No one pushed any hospital to use Toyota Production System (lean) methods. Each hospital was free to innovate.

To everyone's surprise, CLABs were reduced by 68 percent—and the one hospital that fully embraced the TPS/lean method reduced CLABs to zero (a feat that was sustained for years).

The regional collaborative proved that dramatic improvements were possible. Successful hospital units developed standard work, clarified accountability among team members, and collected data and fed it back to the front lines. They began with one significant improvement learned from that experience and translated the learning to solving other problems.

Reduction in Hospital Readmissions for Complex Patients

With support from Center for Medicare and Medicaid Innovation (CMMI), PRHI and six hospital partners opened the first Primary Care Resource Center (PCRC) in 2013. Each PCRC is a support hub, staffed by nurse care managers and pharmacists who improve care and care transitions of complex patients with COPD, heart failure and acute myocardial infarction, thereby reducing avoidable hospitalizations.

Despite substantive clinical guidelines for care of these conditions, effective and systematic implementation of the guidelines remains highly variable. Prior to the CMMI award, PRHI had piloted a PCRC at a regional hospital to create a model incorporating the most important relationships, services, staffing and training methods necessary for the best implementation results.

To spread the model throughout the region, the collaborative needed to enlist the support of leadership at independent regional hospitals—exactly the ones with the smallest profit margins and the fewest resources to adapt to new Medicare and health plan expectations. A strong business case and dedication to using project results to influence payment reform were also critical to leadership adoption of the model. Participating hospitals demonstrated their commitment to the project by supplying space, equipment, capital and support personnel.

The PCRC pilot showed the importance of high-touch care starting during the index hospitalization: PCRC staff members deliver inpatient, as well as post-discharge, care. They see patients multiple times during each admission, including at the point of discharge. They make at least two phone calls post-discharge and conduct home visits to at least a third of patients.

To identify the best mix of care required to lower readmissions, the project used process, outcome and utilization metrics to continually shape the care model rather than imposing a static model on the caregivers. The pilot hospital team learned that successful implementation of evidence-based guidelines requires creativity, experimentation, and attention to the recommendations of staff and patients.

Care managers shared disappointment and frustration at the seemingly low motivation of their complex patients. In addition to strong content from American Heart Association and COPD Foundation, which provided onsite clinical training, educational materials, equipment and continuing education credits, PRHI provided coaching at all sites. Coaching in process improvement, data management and communication skills turned out to be as important as clinical training in cardiopulmonary care.

Shared site visits by each of the PCRC teams enhanced process improvement. Group discussions explored ways to modify workflows. Subsequently, they used PDSA cycles to institute improvements at their own sites.

The PCRC data management and analytics team collaborated with PCRC frontline workers to review the data to help visualize the care outcomes. This did much to increase fidelity and completeness of project data collection. The collaborative nature of these discussions helped frontline staff teach the analytics team about the realities of data collection in the field.

PCRC staff responded enthusiastically to Introduction to Motivational

Interviewing (MI) sessions, which explored a method to elicit the motivation for behavior change through direct communication. Evaluation surveys from participants included comments such as "Using open-ended questions helped me to understand the patient's own life goals and how they related to my advice about smoking cessation. MI techniques allowed me to get a sense of what else was important in their lives and whether those priorities were in conflict."

PRHI responded to PCRC staff requests for more MI training by providing intensive educational opportunities: 90-minute introductory workshop; all-day, indepth workshop with concept discussions, exercises and practice with a simulated patient; booster webinars including sharing of experiences, live polling and homework activities; additional full-day workshop; and, most important, point-of-service coaching. One participant said, "We learned about MI in the classroom, but it wasn't until I saw it demonstrated in real time, with a real patient, with real issues that I realized the impact. I thought I knew how to communicate with patients. The MI coaching noticeably improved my skills."

In its first two years of operation, the PCRC participants reported providing care to more than 6,500 patients, with a reduction in 30-day readmissions by 15.5 percent, and a reduction in total cost of care by 4.3 percent. Staff frustration has given way to cautious but committed optimism.

Medical Home Change Concepts in Smaller Medical Practices

Starting in 2010, PRHI served as a Regional Extension Center, funded through the American Recovery and Reinvestment Act, to assist smaller primary-care medical practices with electronic health records (EHR) implementation. Within four years, more than 750 primary care providers and 260 sites have implemented EHRs successfully.[4] EHR reports allowed providers to examine their own care systematically, exposing some disturbing gaps. At the same time, the payers for healthcare services began to use their claims data to pressure practices to meet external quality, satisfaction and utilization benchmarks. Some health plans began to provide incentives to practices that had achieved medical home status; others even signaled the intent to create favored networks requiring medical home status for membership. However, a typical meeting to urge providers to form Patient Centered Medical Homes would sound like this:

The meeting started promptly at 7:30 a.m. in the basement of the local hospital. Practice managers and physicians from five different offices restlessly checked their cellphones for new tasks being added to an already truncated day. A hospital administrator reminded the provider group that their market share and reimbursement rates would depend on getting certified as Patient Centered Medical Homes (PCMH). The facilitator made it through two slides in the presentation before the medical group director raised his voice, "You know, you people from the health plans and the government are driving us crazy with one program after another claiming to improve quality and save money, and all they do is slow me down and cost me money."

The flood of forms, expectations, threats and disincentives has created a siege mentality in medical practices, especially those with little or no administrative reserve. Telling this audience more about PCMH was going to be a waste of time.

Instead our Medical Home trainer said, "Thanks for coming in for the meeting this morning. I know you have a busy day ahead. And that's why we're here. We've seen the pressures mounting on smaller practices such as yours. We know that you became nurses and doctors to give the very best care possible. We're here to work with you to overcome the barriers to giving that kind of care. Tell us what issues you're facing. I'll write them up here on the whiteboard."

As each problem was mentioned, the associated goal was placed next to it on the board. Soon there was a map of the practice leadership's goals and the obstacles they encountered in meeting those goals.

This technique models an important organizational process for practices, while fulfilling the need for leadership involvement and direction. This is motivational interviewing directed toward leadership engagement—participants safely share realities, challenges and dreams to create the foundation for practice transformation.

A participant said, "At the first meeting, participants started the process of identifying the goals of their practices. At the last meeting they mapped out the work that would be required to provide the care a complex patient would really need to achieve optimum goals. They identified work to be done before, during and after the office visit. Since that session, they met with other providers and staff in their practices to make sure they didn't leave anything out. I asked, 'What did you learn?' One of the front desk supervisors looked grim and said that the doctor tried to do all the diabetes things listed, but got so far behind that three of his patients had to be rescheduled at the end of the day."

During the robust discussion that followed, members of each of the practices chimed in with anecdotes and observations about their own attempts to institute change: "You can't just start doing something new. It affects everybody in the office. You need to all work on this together." They all agreed that they needed help in figuring out which changes to make and when.

They had all come to the conclusion independently that a process improvement team was necessary. While these practices differed in size, staffing and organization, they began to develop a sense of their common journey through these working meetings. They began to take advantage of the diversity of experience in the group to seek out new ideas and perspectives. Several of the practice teams exchanged phone numbers to arrange site visits.

The project team realized that they were now ready to accept coaching. PRHI scheduled on-site visits with each practice to support team formation, with the added goal of modeling an effective process-improvement meeting.

Behavioral Care Integrated into Primary Care Practices

The COMPASS program, Care of Mental, Physical and Substance Use Syndromes, is a team-based healthcare model that promotes evidence-based behavioral healthcare in primary care settings to treat patients suffering from depression, in addition to diabetes or cardiovascular disease. As one of eight national partners for the CMMI-funded project, PRHI provided training and coaching to practices to help them implement a collaborative care model that includes systematic treatment to outcome targets, weekly case review and dedicated care management.

While recruiting practices for the project, participants often stated, "We have enough trouble taking care of medical illnesses without adding depression to the list." PRHI sat down with clinical leaders to review their practice data. It demonstrated the system's failure to effectively control risks associated with diabetes, high cholesterol and hypertension. During a root-cause analysis exercise, the practice leaders progressively identified critical logistic, social, environmental and behavioral issues that trump the impact of the medical care they provide to their patients. "If COMPASS can help with these issues, sign me up," they said.

Thirty-one primary care practices in three practice networks committed to implementing COMPASS and began the process of recruiting and training care managers, mostly registered nurses transitioning from the acute setting. They needed orientation not only for behavioral health issues but also for communication styles, community resources and the chronic care model.

Consulting medical and psychiatric consultants were identified to work with the care managers each week in systematic case review sessions. They too found themselves in uncharted territory.

In spite of carefully wrought, multi-disciplinary training at the onset of the project, including patient simulators, participants struggled with applying their learning in context.

"COMPASS was added on top of our existing work. During the training, I was in a fog and didn't fully understand what it was. We couldn't see how it fit into our traditional care management work back in the office," they said.

The coaches decided to accompany care managers during office and telephone contacts and in case-review meetings to mentor effective use of motivational interviewing and behavioral activation.

The nurse care managers needed a chance to reflect on their conversations with patients. They were amazed at what they learned by asking open-ended questions. But they feared being stuck on the phone forever or hearing about problems they couldn't deal with effectively. Talking with the coach, they could think through a better conversation the next time. Some of the care managers found it helpful to call our coaches after difficult encounters.

As coaching support created greater confidence, care managers boosted their patient contact rates, improved the quality of collaboration with consultants and enhanced patients' self-care success. Regular webinars and phone conferences provided opportunities for sharing across corporate and state borders.

One of the care managers said, "I thought the COMPASS webinars helped because you often feel alone. They gave me knowledge about what other people are doing and how they were solving their problems. COMPASS itself grew as we went along and discovered how to do things better. It was fun!"

This is a critical role of collaboratives: Group participation creates a community of shared interest, common identity and mutual commitment. Above all, they create motivated change agents. Each practice network began to see the leadership potential in their COMPASS care managers, and they began to use them to train others in the collaborative care model. Care manager champions emerged and took on responsibility for reviewing operational and clinical data, running root-cause analysis sessions and providing coaching in quality improvement and MI.

Conclusion

Knowledge is only one of the precursors to action; effective educational techniques incorporate methods that encourage organizational development. Although project, grant and contract deliverables remain important, successful facilitators put the participant's and ultimately the patient's and family's needs first. This requires that trainers and facilitators are not only participant-centered but actually participant-directed, to enable practices and organizations to make changes required to accelerate improvement to meet the new expectations of accountable care.

Content expertise has its greatest impact when combined with process improvement and communication skills development. Desired behavior change could not be achieved without opportunities for exploration through shadowing, simulation, collaborative discussion and in-context coaching.

Sustained change requires alignment of incentives, provision of adequate staffing and resources, and grooming of embedded champions to continue the iterative steps toward perfect patient care. These champions create wider and wider networks of people committed to change. To not endorse a worthy improvement is soon regarded as being indifferent to progress. Ideas begin to self-propel. This is the key to sustainable organizational improvement. As the PRHI CEO says to every fellowship class or champions learning collective: "You think I regard you simply as students of quality improvement. But I believe I'm looking at the army of the quality revolution."

[1] *Pro-Change Behavior Systems, Inc.* (2014). Retrieved from The transtheoretical Model (TTM): http://www.prochange.com/

[2] Leape, L. (1994). Error in medicine. *JAMA , 272* (73), 1851-7.

[3] Leape, L. (2014, Nov). PRHI Executive Summary & Data. *Pittsburgh Regional Health Initiative & Jewish Healthcare Foundation*

[4] Block, B. (2010). *The Regional Extension and Assistance Center for Health Information Technology in Western Pennsylvania (REACH)*. Retrieved from Pittsburgh Regional Health Initiative: http://www.prhi.org/initiatives/reach

CHAPTER 11

Optimizing Data and Measurement: Just Enough Data for Success

By Sam R. Watson, MSA, CPPS and Deneil LoGiudice
Collaborative Public Reporting by Jim Chase Understanding the
Best Way to Display Data to Meet Your Goals by Jason Byrd, J.D.

"Lies, damn lies and statistics."

—Mark Twain

Introduction

Data is the fuel that feeds the engine of improvement. If data is incomplete, inaccurate, or burdensome or measuring the wrong thing, the improvement engine will fail to function properly.

During the improvement process, data makes it possible to progress toward and achieve your intended goals. Making a plan that will guide you through the requirements of data collection will help you determine the validity, feasibility, reliability, quantity and frequency of the data measures. Analyzing the data will help determine the need for action. And stakeholder participation will nurture ownership and sustainability of the system.

Measurement Planning

"If you don't know how to ask the right question, you discover nothing."
—W. Edwards Deming

When planning a collaborative, data planning is paramount. The first step in data planning is to determine the aim, or aims. The aims lead to the intended outcome of a given intervention.[1] As a plan for improvement is developed, a hypothesis, either formal or informal, is put forward. The hypothesis forms the foundation for the data collection and measurement strategy.

When developing this strategy, it's helpful to turn to the model of care offered by physician and health services researcher Avedis Donabedian that considers three elements of measurement: structure, process and outcome.[2] Let's apply this model to the following example:

The aim is to reduce the rate of *Clostridium difficile (C. difficile)* bacterium infection by 25 percent. A hypothesis is that implementing a hand hygiene protocol will reduce the rate of *C. difficile* infection. The outcome measure rate of *C. difficile* is self-evident, but what about the structure and process? The amount of hand cleaner that is consumed is a possible process measure of the performance of hand hygiene. The number and placement of sinks and hand-cleaner dispensers is a structural measure.

All three measures in this example—structure, process and outcome— demonstrate the success or failure of the hypothesis that supports the overall aim. The structural measure identifies barriers to hand hygiene. The process measure demonstrates compliance with hand hygiene. And the *C. difficile* infection rate reflects the outcome related to the use of hand hygiene.

Data Capture Method

Once the measures have been identified, the next step in the data collection plan is to determine how the data may be captured. A survey of potential data sources should consider existing as well as *de novo* collection. Data could be culled from existing data sources such as medical, laboratory, pharmacy or financial records.

A data collection tool will need to be developed for *de novo* data. This tool can be as simple as a tally sheet for counts, or more developed, such as an electronic spreadsheet or database. Other potential data collection methods include surveys, interviews, forms and direct observation.

Don't let perfection be the enemy of good. Consider following the software development concept of minimum viable product (MVP): Even if a product has known bugs, it still works and meets the minimum requirements.[3] The shortcomings are outweighed by the importance of getting the product into the hands of users, getting feedback and incorporating the needed updates. Releasing an MVP enables the plan-do-check-act loop to start with minimal amount of effort and least amount of development time upfront (Figure 1).

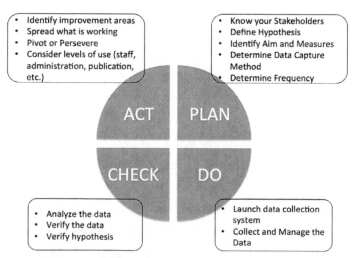

Figure 1. The plan-do-check-act approach can be applied when developing and deploying a data measurement system.

In data management, the product is the data collection system or method, such as a simple tally sheet kept by an admissions person. After testing the tally sheet method, you can incorporate feedback and improvement suggestions to improve the data collection.

Key Elements of a Measurement Plan

Regardless of the source of the data, preparation of the data collection plan should include a number of considerations. First, key stakeholders of the system should participate in the design of the data collection plan when possible. This will promote buy-in, ownership and support, strengthening the system and improving its sustainability.

Second, you should address these key elements of a measurement plan:

- Validity
- Feasibility
- Reliability
- Quantity
- Frequency
- Metrics definition
- Quality checks

Validity

When selecting measures, a literature review for an intervention should include a review for measure recommendations. For example, look to the Centers for Disease Control and Prevention for a standardized measure used for *C. difficile*.

Feasibility

When planning measures, consider feasibility. A measure may have a strong relationship to an intervention but may be too burdensome to collect. Evaluate the resources required to consistently and accurately collect the data.

Elaborate data collection and analysis systems often become cumbersome and people stop using them. Knowing who will enter and use the data and the environment in which this takes place will influence the design of the system. For example, if the point of data entry is removed from a computer, you may need an alternative collection method such as a mobile device or pen and paper. On the other hand, if the data is directly captured in the lab reporting system via data export, no data entry person is needed. Collaboratives may use other data-entry techniques that include a password-protected web portal or compatible spreadsheets/workbooks or databases.

Reliability

When testing measures, you should consider the reliability of collecting the data according to the measure specifications (e.g., numerator and denominator definitions). Additionally, running a test of the data collection will help to determine if training is needed to collect the data. It will also help to identify unpredicted barriers and, if necessary, test inter-rater reliability, that is, data collected consistently across multiple data collectors. Testing inter-rater reliability is an important consideration if there's intent to publish.

As part of the testing, it's important to determine if there's a need to train data collectors on the use of the instrument. If so, it becomes part of the collection and management plan.

Quantity

It's important to stick to only the "vital few" measures. If there are too many measures, it can have a negative effect, diverting focus from what's being improved.

Ultimately, this could lead to a greater risk of incomplete or erroneous data, or lack of sustainability.

At the same time, if a measure is too simplistic, it may not provide sufficient data to answer the hypothesis. It's helpful to think of measures on a continuum of scientific soundness that's supported by literature and feasibility (Figure 2).[4]

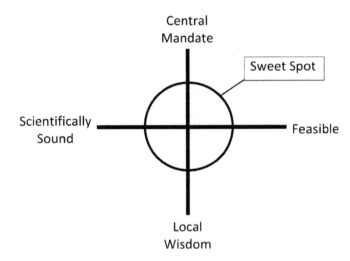

Figure 2. Find the sweet spot between scientifically sound and feasible measures.

Finding the balance between the two ends of the measure spectrum will yield a greater likelihood of complete and meaningful data. Taking into account local wisdom to inform measure selection may increase support for collection and derive greater meaning.

The quantity of measures collected at the collaborative level may differ from the amount of measures collected at the facility. The measures that need to be centrally reported should tie to the overall aim of the collaborative, such as with the C. difficile infection rate, where process or structural measures used to answer the hypothesis may only be tracked at the participating facility.

Frequency

Determining the baseline period and frequency of data collection depends, in part, on the frequency of what's being measured. In the C. *difficile* example, with a high number of cases, say, eight to 10 per month, a shorter baseline may be sufficient. However, if the occurrences are rare, one or less per month, a longer baseline may be necessary to gain enough analytical power to determine statistical significance.

In addition to the need to assure sufficient data for analysis, it's important to consider the frequency of feedback to the improvement team. For example, quarterly is often not enough. Even if numbers are small, more frequent collection is important, and the analysis for significance can be done once a sufficient data set is collected. The frequency of collection must match the need as outlined in the plan.

Sampling is helpful to reduce the burden of data collection and also depends on the frequency of measurement. This can be determined if the number of instances being measured is high enough. There's no need to capture every event to allow for sufficient analysis. Sampling strategies are beyond the scope of this book; however, there are a number of methods, including simplistic randomization, which is easily done with a random number generator in a spreadsheet program.

There are other considerations that should be accounted for in the collection and analysis of the data, such as seasonality or significant events (e.g., seasonal outbreaks, disaster response, etc.).

Metrics Definition

Once the measures are determined, you should incorporate them into a data dictionary. Those collecting and analyzing the data must understand the definitions. The data dictionary contains the pertinent information about a measure, including source, type of measures (e.g., structural, process and outcome), inclusions and exclusions, and frequency (Table 1).

Measure	Collection Year	Source	Variable	Type	Measure Names	Numerators and Denominators	Inclusions	Exclusions	Collection Schedule
Adverse Drug Events	2014	Excel Spreadsheet	o1	Outcome	(Insulin) Percent of inpatient blood glucose levels < 40 mg/dl	Numerator: number of inpatient blood glucose levels < 40 mg/dl	All inpatients have had a blood glucose during an inpatient admission.		Monthly
						Denominator: number of inpatient blood glucose levels measured			
Adverse Drug Events	2014	Excel spreadsheet	o2	Outcome	(Anticoagulant) Percent of inpatients on warfarin with an INR level >5	Numerator: number of inpatient INR levels >5	All inpatients have had an INR drawn during an inpatient visit.		Monthly
						Denominator: number of inpatient INR levels measured			

Table 1. Example data for two types of adverse drug events

Quality Checks

Conduct data quality checks to detect if data is accurate and complete and collected as planned. Quality checks may identify one or more data issues, including but not limited to the following:

- Inaccurate data
- Missing or incomplete data
- Falsified or manipulated data
- Challenges with collecting the data, such as the only person who knows how to collect the data is on vacation

If any of these challenges are identified, corrective measures should be implemented immediately. Additional audits may be necessary to ensure the issues are resolved.

Quality checks could be built into the software or the spreadsheet, or conducted through audits. One example of a quality check is to randomly select a data collection form and audit the data to check for completeness, any outliers or astronomical data points. These might actually be typos and should be investigated and understood. Another form of a quality check is to set up

201

the collection spreadsheet to not allow unrealistic numbers, such as a negative number for blood pressure. To verify that the measurement tool is understood, you could ask multiple people to step through the data collection steps and compare results among them. If the results don't match, investigate why.

You can also make quality checks at the level of the entire collaborative. Dramatically changing denominators, zero/zero entries or empty fields may be a sign of data issues.

You should mitigate the risk of missing data during the data collection planning process and the testing of the data collection tools. However, during live collection, there are unforeseen occurrences that may result in incomplete data. Monitoring data during the collection is imperative to ensure there are no gaps. To make sure data is as complete as possible, ask data collectors about any missing data and address barriers or unexpected issues.

Project Plan Submission

Some projects require institutional review board (IRB) approval. This review may be appropriate if there's intent to publish or generalize knowledge you gain from an initiative.[5] Additionally, it may be appropriate to consider an IRB if there are privacy or security concerns with the data. http://www.fda.gov/RegulatoryInformation/Guidances/ucm126420.htm is a useful website to learn more about IRBs.

Key Themes

- Determine what data you need to collect to meet the goal.
- Consider using the Donabedian model of structure, process and outcome.
- Evaluate measure characteristics, including validity, feasibility, reliability, quantity and frequency.

- Test measures before fully deploying.
- Develop a data dictionary that contains the pertinent information about the measures.

Case Study: Collaborative Public Reporting

Jim Chase and Gail Amundson, M.D.

It takes a community to transform healthcare. And "measures that matter" are necessary to do just that. Measures that matter are clinically relevant measures that effectively highlight large gaps in care and stimulate deep systematic change that leads to leaps in the quality of healthcare.

MN Community Measurement (MNCM) is a pioneering non-profit organization that is contributing to these leaps by developing measures, collecting comparable data across health systems and reporting it publicly. It began in 2000, when three medical directors of the largest health plans in Minnesota began laying the groundwork for a common reporting system that would stimulate faster and greater improvements in patient care than existing separate reporting systems.

The environment was ripe for such an effort. At the time, health plan quality measurement in Minnesota was extremely burdensome. For diabetes measures alone, 12,000 records were reviewed in the year before MNCM's founding.[6] A more sophisticated sampling method would greatly reduce the number of patient records needing review and, importantly, provide reliable data on provider practices. Extensive public reporting of health plan performance was demonstrating only small differences in quality despite the knowledge of large differences in quality among provider practices.

With its steering committee comprised of practice leaders and health plan medical directors, help from Minnesota Council of Health Plans, and Minnesota Medical Association as a supporting member, MNCM was launched. Critically, the aspirational *Healthcare Effectiveness Data and Information Set* (HEDIS)-based Optimal Diabetes Care measure was the first piloted by the group. A composite measure of diabetes care from the perspective of individual patients, it asks the question, "Did this patient reach all guideline-recommended treatment targets for modifying cardiovascular risk?" At the time, those targets were controlling blood pressure, LDL cholesterol and A1C; avoiding smoking; and taking aspirin daily. Each could also be measured individually.

Despite excellent rates for individual measures, the number of patients meeting all treatment targets was quite low.[7] In some practices, no patients met all targets. "All-or-none" optimal care measures clearly indicated the continuing opportunity to improve patient care. With public reporting on the line, and health plan incentives aligned behind the results, practices had the reason they needed to tackle the exceptionally difficult but essential task of redesigning patient care processes to achieve better results.

The systems focus stimulated by optimal care measures has paid off. For example, compared to static national anti-platelet prophylaxis rates that are below 50 percent, Minnesota anti-platelet prophylaxis averages 95 percent, with many practices achieving rates of 100 percent.[8] Minnesota has the lowest death rate from heart disease in the country, and there is no disparity in death rate from heart disease between African-Americans and the overall population as there is nationally.

Using aspirational composite measures is central to the success of MNCM, measures that align with locally accepted guideline recommendations and resonate as clinically relevant with clinicians.

Testing and Deployment

Once those participating document and understand the measurement plan elements, the data collection system is ready to launch.

Prototype

Select a small group of stakeholders for a prototype of the data collection. Start with a data collection tool, get feedback and incorporate it into the next iteration. Continue this process until the system works well. As in the previous example of the MVP, stick to a short time frame and use the value of real-time feedback to improve the system as you go along. There's no need to wait for a robust system with all the bells and whistles when a piece of paper and a pen will work. Don't let perfection be the enemy of good.

Training

Train the participants in the data collection. This could be done in advance or in real time, during the launch. Training may take different forms (e.g., written documentation, webinars or demonstrations), depending on the complexity of the data collection tool. At the collaborative, maintain a list of data contacts for each participating organization.

Feedback and Review

A constant and continuous feedback loop on data capture will ensure you can quickly change the collection methods or measures if needed. Feedback should focus on the topics previously discussed in the "Key Elements of a Measurement Plan" section, including data collection frequency and quality.

Real-time feedback review can allow for modifications to the system, process or structure, such as correcting a survey question that isn't clear.

Spend time with the users of the data collection system in the place where the data collection activities and process improvement take place. This will help give you a better understanding of any potential barriers and possibly expedite the improvement process while building rapport with the people directly involved, strengthening the quality and quantity of feedback.

Key Themes

- Launch the data collection system using a methodological approach including pilot testing and feedback.
- Train the data collection participants in the data plan.
- Use the value of real-time feedback to improve the system as you go along.

Analysis, Display and Use of Data

"If the statistics are boring, then you've got the wrong numbers."
—Edward Tufte

"The temptation to form premature theories upon insufficient data is the bane of our profession."
—Sherlock Holmes

Data should be our friend. How we analyze, display and utilize data is a key factor in making it the friend of those who can impact the change we are seeking.

Objective

Knowing the objective of the data collection (adherence to standards, quality control, improvement or publication) will inform how to display and use the data. When used for adherence or quality control, the objective is to ensure consistent performance in the process and identify variation in the process so you can make corrections before a standard violation occurs. When using data for improvement, the objective is to identify patterns in the data. These patterns will help highlight where improvement is needed, where interventions or small tests are making a difference, and whether the improvement is sustaining and what improvements are ready to scale.

Current performance compared to benchmarks, as well as shifts or trends, will indicate if action is required. One benefit of being part of a collaborative is that an organization can use feedback and comparative data from the other organizations in the collaborative to make improvements.

Data for research and publication may use data plots, such as box plots, to demonstrate outliers, or scatter plots to show correlation.

Audience

In addition to knowing the objective of the data collection, you must know the audience or those using the data. It's likely that you will have multiple audiences for the data you collect, so you may be required to report the data in multiple formats. At the end of the day, you want to display your data in such a way that it's easy to interpret and will trigger action.

Let's revisit the C. *difficile* example. In this case, there most likely will be multiple audiences who will utilize the data. One group might be the clinical staff, another might be the administrative staff and a third might be a collaborative. The clinical staff can directly influence the process measure: adherence to hand hygiene. So the best data to review with them would be the amount of hand cleaner consumed.

Understanding the Best Way to Display Data to Meet Your Goals

By Jason Byrd, J.D.

Driving meaningful improvement requires appropriate data and valid understanding and interpretation of that data. So displaying the data effectively is critical.

The old adage, "A picture says a thousand words," can often apply to uses of data to drive improvement. Carolinas HealthCare System, a Hospital Engagement Network (HEN), selected to help reduce harm and improve patient care and safety among its facilities, learned that the most effective data strategy properly balances standardized and customized approaches.

Standardized approaches include scorecards, where a legend, color scheme and display are used to provide common understandings and comparisons. These scorecards provide structure, data definitions and ease to quickly identify improvement opportunities. As part of its HEN efforts, Carolinas HealthCare System uses facility-specific scorecards that easily identify each measure's baseline and performance (rates, numerators, denominators), using a color scheme to easily identify performance relative to harm reduction goals.

While the standardized approach is generally effective at one level, flexibility is required to drive improvements at some facilities. For example, at one of Carolinas HealthCare System's facilities, the team spent a significant amount of time debating the usefulness of rates on certain lower volume metrics.

The administrative staff and upper management may be more interested in the outcome measure, the cost of care, the structure measures and, ultimately, the rate of *C. difficile* infection. The collaborative is using this data to understand if it is reaching its aim in aggregate and what, if any, organizations are struggling and might need additional support.

Visualization and Display

Once you know the objective and specific audience, you can determine the appropriate and most effective data visualization. Unless your audience are data analysts, avoid displaying data in tables or crowded spreadsheets. Data is more meaningful when it's displayed visually.

Effective data visualization increases the power of communication. It's important to remember that data is one form of information. Sometimes very simple descriptions of data are the most powerful motivators. For example, using names (or partially de-identified names) of patients who died from specific complications instead of abstract numbers (e.g., total number of deaths) is more effective in communicating that these are real people who may have died unnecessarily. Another example is using the number of days between events. While there are advanced statistical methods to determine the significance of the number of days between certain events, most staff intuitively know, with no additional information, that a larger number of days between events is the goal, or aim. A score sheet showing the number of days since the last event is a very good friend indeed.

Run Charts

There are a number of tools for displaying and analyzing collected data. Perhaps the simplest is the run chart, which plots the variable being measured against a time series (Figure 3). Run charts allow simple visual inspection to identify trends in the data. This is an effective tool for sharing with the improvement teams.

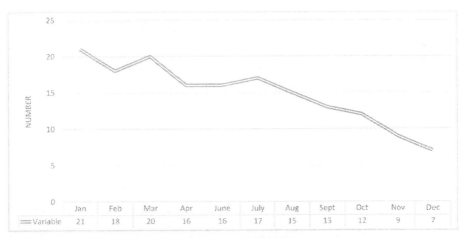

	Jan	Feb	Mar	Apr	June	July	Aug	Sept	Oct	Nov	Dec
═══ Variable	21	18	20	16	16	17	15	13	12	9	7

Figure 3. Example run chart showing a variable against a timeline.

Knowing and tracking data at frequent intervals tells a more accurate story and provides insight into the effectiveness of the intervention.

But by transitioning to displaying the number of patients harmed each month, the hospital was able to hold productive discussions about each improvement area.

Some facilities want to understand their performance in relation to national or regional benchmarks; some want comparisons to local prominent organizations; while others want to be the best within their system or HEN. Understanding these cultural dynamics and displaying the data appropriately are essential to triggering local action.

To understand what this means in regard to the overall progress, a goal line is often added to the chart. The goal line makes the data more tangible and helps explain its meaning. A trajectory line will further demonstrate what the data is telling us. It can tell us if we are on target to meet our end goal and how much further we have to go (Figure 4).[9]

The example in Figure 4 tracks the data at a frequency that supports the speed of change. The results are timely, monthly rather than annual, and avoid historical numbers. In addition, effort is made to get this data to the improvement teams on a weekly basis to expedite the improvement process.

Next, the target is known, and current performance is tracked in relation to the goal. The example tracks the monthly placement rate against the target monthly placement rate. Note that the actual monthly placement rate changes each month based on the previous month's rate. Therefore, in months where the target is not met, the next month goal increases to make up for the gap.

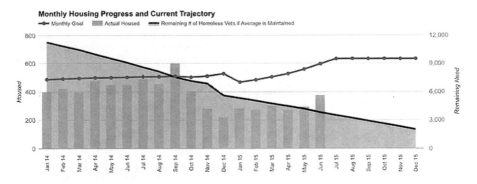

Figure 4. Trajectory line shows how close United Way of Los Angeles is to its goal of ending veteran homelessness by the end of 2015.

Additionally, the trajectory line shows that if the system continues to perform at the same monthly placement rate, there will still be nearly 3,000 homeless veterans by the end of the targeted timeline.[10]

Trend lines should be used with caution. Trends need to meet specific criteria, and some software may suggest a trend when in fact no trend is actually present. A trend may also cause staff to "let off the gas," assuming they are on a trajectory to success. But noting a trend may be helpful if you are trying to accelerate the rate of improvement (e.g., hitting your target on time at the current rate of improvement).

Statistical Process Control

In a more advanced approach, you can apply statistical process control (SPC) with a data set to determine variation. With SPC, a chart uses a time series and also includes upper and lower control limits based on mean and standard deviation (Figure 5). By using the control limits, the analysis can determine whether the variation is due to common cause or special cause.[11]

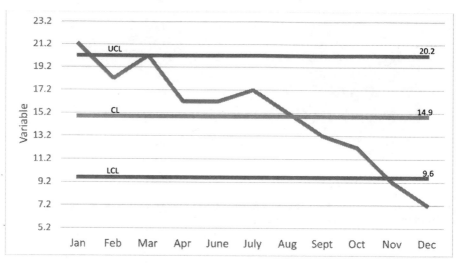

Figure 5. Statistical process control chart includes upper and lower control limits based on mean and standard deviation.

Common cause variation is the result of normal variation. For example, temperatures during a season may vary in a given region. Historical records make this variability evident. Say you are in the Midwest and the temperatures during winter range from zero to the mid-30s. Looking back over several years of meteorological records, you could apply SPC to the data with control limits, and you would see this pattern of variability, barring any unusual meteorological activity.

Special cause variation comes into play when there is variation outside of the predicted range. In the Midwest temperature example, if a polar vortex causes the temperature to fall into the subzero range for a period of time, it would be special cause variation.

Recognizing these types of variations is important when trying to understand the impact of an intervention. Looking back to our running example of improving hand hygiene to reduce *C. difficile* infection, we notice that after analyzing the consumption of soap after implementing a hand hygiene protocol, the use of hand soap increases above the normal rate. A possible conclusion is the intervention was successful in increasing hand hygiene. Keeping the hypothesis in mind, the next question should be: Is the special cause variation in the use of hand hygiene resulting in a decreasing *C. difficile* infection rate?

Leading and Lagging Indicators

In quality improvement, we often refer to process and outcome measures. This is an appropriate time to consider leading and lagging indicators. Process measures may be considered leading indicators; that is, they most often change (positive or negative) in advance of the outcome, or lagging indicator (Table 2). In the *C. difficile* example, while we may see an increase in the use of hand hygiene, the infection rate may not yet show a decrease. This is a result of the process measure serving as a leading indicator. In other words, this rate may change in advance of the outcome measure (*C. difficile* infection rate), which would be the lagging indicator.

Leading Indicator/Process Measure	Lagging Indicator/Outcome Measure
Adherence to surgical sponge count	Retained foreign object
Fluid bolus for resuscitation of severe shock	Decreased mortality in patients with a diagnosis of shock
Improvement in the use of a central-line-placement checklist	Reduced central-line-associated bloodstream infections

Table 2. Examples of process and outcome measures with leading and lagging indicators

Once the data from the lagging indicator "catches up," you can evaluate whether a change in the leading indicator has resulted in a change in the lagging measure. If the analysis of the *C. difficile* rate using SPC shows a concomitant special cause variation, where the infections are decreasing, it may reflect the result of improved hand hygiene.

If there's interest in publishing the results of the improvement effort, determine whether there are other factors, sometimes referred to as "secular influences," that may also have an effect on the change. This would require comparing the results of the data collected during the intervention to a control group.

What this also means is that if data doesn't suggest you're achieving your goal, some questions should be asked at the organizational or collaborative level:

- Are the measures the correct measures? If not, why not? What measures should be tracked? Give permission to abandon measures if they are not helping.
- Is the frequency adequate? Does it give enough time to respond to either improve or maintain standards?
- Is data tracked consistently? Where are the gaps and why?
- Is data displayed in a manner that is useful to the audience or user?
- Is the process clearly linked to the outcome? If so, are other factors overwhelming any improvement in the overall outcome?

The overall objective is to make the data tangible and meaningful to your audience. If we make data our friend, it will help us achieve our objective, whether that be for quality improvement, control or publication.

Key Themes

- Know the objective and audience.
- Make data visual. For some audiences, data tables are effective, but most need a graphical display.
- Adding target and trajectory lines may help demonstrate progress.
- Run charts are a basic yet powerful tool to display and analyze data trends and shifts.
- SPC charts are an effective means of determining variation.
- Identify leading and lagging indicators.

Conclusion

Throughout the improvement process, data is an important means to assure the effort is progressing and achieving the intended aims:

- Plan for data collection.
- Tie into the aims that you seek to achieve.
- Consider the validity, feasibility, reliability, quantity and frequency of measures.
- Before collection begins, engage the process stakeholders to help guide the requirements for data collection.
- Deploy the data collection plan methodically.
- Determine the most effective means to share the data. Effective data display provides feedback to the stakeholders.
- Analyze data using basic run charts or more advanced methods such as SPC analysis to determine the need for action.

---

[1] Needham, D., Sinopoli, D., Dinglas, V., Berenholtz, S., Korupolu, R., Watson, S., et al. (2009). Improving data quality control in quality improvement projects. *Int. J Qual Health Care* , 21 (2), 145-50.

[2] Donabedian, A. (1988). The Quality of Care: How Can It Be Assessed. *JAMA* , 260 (12), 1743-1748.

[3] Ries, E. (2011). The Lean Startup: How Today's Entrepreneurs Use Continuous Improvement to Create Radically Successful Businesses. *Crown Business* , 93-113.

[4] Pronovost, P., personal communication.

[5] Protection of Human Subjects, 46 CFR, SS46.101 (2009). (n.d.).

[6] (2012). *Minnesota Death rate from heart disease same for African American and White:*. Minnesota Department of Health & Healthy Minnesota Partnership , Saint Paul, MN.

[7] Number of Heart Disease Deaths per 100,000 Population by Gender. (2015). *Data* . The Henry J. Kaiser Family Foundation.

[8] Prarek, & al., e. (2013, Jan 17). National Antiplatelet use rate. *New England Journal of Medicine* .

[9] *Monthly Housing Project and Current Trajectory*. (2015, June 26). Retrieved from United Way of Greater Los Angeles County: http://hacollab.weebly.com/ending-veteran-homelessness.html

[10] *Current homeless count results*. (n.d.). Retrieved from Los Angeles Homeless Services Authority: http://www.lahsa.org/homelesscount_results

[11] Walton, M. (1986). *The Deming Managment Method*. New York: Perigee Book by The Berkely Publishing Group.

CHAPTER 12

Engaging and Activating Patients and Families

By Karen Wolk Feinstein, Ph.D. and Nancy D. Zionts, MBA
The Hoy Family Story by Libby Hoy
A Spark that Ignited an Entire Organization by Jim Conway, MS, LFACHE

Editor's note: Much of All In: Using Healthcare Collaboratives to Save Lives and Improve Care is oriented to large-scale and enduring learning networks of various stakeholders, often attempting to spread effective practices among different healthcare providers. This chapter also examines more ad hoc types of shared learning experiences where people associate towards a common goal to accelerate the exchange of knowledge, techniques, practices or advocacy. Principles of design are often similar to those described in previous chapters, but in this case are often stimulated, led or conducted by patients, families or the broad category of consumers.

Introduction

Efforts to improve the quality, safety and efficiency of U.S. healthcare for the past 20 years have tested myriad possible solutions—from "lean" and efficiency-driven systems management to performance measurement and public reporting to payment and practice reforms. There have been successes,

A Spark that Ignited an Entire Organization

By Jim Conway, MS, LFACHE.

Our collective and individual burden at Dana-Farber Cancer Institute (DFCI) in 1995 was enormous. Betsy Lehman died after a preventable error: a fourfold overdose of chemotherapy. Our responsibility was clear: Build a culture and set in place the systems that would prevent such an event from ever happening again.

The journey had to be grounded in partnership with patients and families. Betsy thought there was something wrong and we didn't listen to her. We now had to show we honor the voices of all of our patients and their family members. At previous leadership positions in pediatrics, a number of our leaders had experienced the powerful impact of family partnership and thought the same potential in adult cancer care was enormous.

In 1996, the governing board and executive leadership of DFCI made patient and family-centered care a priority and set the expectation that patients and family members would populate all decision-making bodies and structures of the organization.[1] This wasn't an "if," but a "when, where and how" discussion. Staff with long-smoldering ideas for partnership enthusiastically jumped in with dreams of resource centers, patient education materials, patient experience surveys, pain management and more.

We needed to position staff, as well as patients and family members, for success. We sought advice from Institute for Patient- and Family-Centered Care. To signal and ensure accountability at every level, patients and family members also joined the

but too few. Each intervention was trialed in a seriously flawed market in which buyers of healthcare (employers and consumers) blindly negotiated for value—usually through insurance intermediaries. Purchasers seek access to the safest and most reliable providers at the lowest cost without reliable information on either cost or quality.

Mrs. Jones, 75, goes to her medical visit with a traditional perspective. She relies on her doctor to fix her aches and ensure her health. She also relies on her doctor to tell her what's wrong with her, why she feels pain or illness, what tests will confirm this, what medication and treatment options are best for her, and when she should return for another visit. Her granddaughter Lucy, on the other hand, a 24-year-old accountant, approaches her physician differently. She's already investigated possible causes of her discomfort on a host of Internet sites, considered the most likely source, reviewed the treatment options, and considered the side effects of any potential medications and the risk/ gain from doing various diagnostic tests.

She's aware of what tests and interventions are evidence-based and which are contraindicated by credible sources. Lucy communicates with her doctor by email, they concur on next steps, and Lucy concludes by saying that she'll revisit the situation if the immediate remedy isn't successful.

It's possible that patients like Lucy will forever change medicine. They may be the lever that finally contains costs and produces a healthier population. Lucy is taking responsibility for her health. She sets her own health goals and adjusts her lifestyle to achieve them. She gathers information on various providers and is an informed "health shopper."

Patient and family activation has risen to the top of the list of key strategies for health reformers. And we're not talking about adherence, inclusion or compliance. This new era of true patient activation envisions a *fundamental realignment* of patient and provider roles and responsibilities, where patients create new connections and take charge of their decisions, care and health. And the millennials may well represent the first generation who, as a whole, have come to regard their health as their responsibility. They're skeptical about medicine's capability to perform magic fixes and about their motivations and currency.

This generation will insist that the health settings from which they receive care provide respect and courtesy; if not, the activated patients will express their preferences, get satisfaction or find another provider. Activated patients as consumers are not "empowered" by anyone but themselves to play the major role in their care and decision-making; it comes from within. Activated patients therefore cannot be described as compliant because they own their treatment options and actions; following orders is not in the game plan. They'll demand the information they need to be smart shoppers and self-managers. In addition, collaboratives that don't engage with consumers, don't accommodate changing preferences and behaviors, and don't actively solicit suggestions from consumers could develop ineffective or suboptimal strategies.

This chapter provides an overview of the forces underlying what we call the "patient activation movement."

Center's Governing Board table.

The power of this partnership immediately revealed the bumpy care continuum of our patients, the gap between what we say and do, the seemingly endless learning of things we didn't know but patients and families did, for example. As the journey continued, it was matched with great wisdom, the collective pride in collaborative practice, continuous improvement and sustained outcomes. Susan M. Grant, MS, RN, chief nursing officer, after listening to powerful input during one of the first meetings with patients and family members, said, "We will never be the same again."[2] We weren't and that was great!

Why the Shift?

The past decades have witnessed a "flattening of expert hierarchies." People are less likely to trust expert opinion. Advocacy movements such as "nothing about me without me" call for the creation of "participatory medicine." More recently, Pew Research Center studies on millennials document a widespread distrust of medical establishment practices and the financial motives behind various treatment recommendations.[3] There's not a single driving force behind the shift to patient activation. A combination of developments from technological advances to policy change allow consumers unprecedented access to information.

The health professionals gathered at the headquarters of AARP in Washington, D.C., in 2010 were intrigued with their summons to this unusual and unexpected event. In effect, here was "half a Noah's ark," one of just about every stakeholder in the healthcare galaxy and a myriad of policy rainmakers. They spent a day considering how to build consumer and physician consensus around payment reform. This ad hoc collaborative accomplished a great deal in seven hours. The impact of their gathering has been impressive.

Affordable Care Act

The breadth of the 2010 Patient Protection and Affordable Care Act (ACA) is profound. It gave the "awakening" of consumer-directed and focused healthcare more than a shot in the arm; it gave it a new body, a jaw and teeth. The ACA shepherds in new roles for consumers. Millions now have access to insurance and healthcare for the first time. Moreover, ACA reforms related to transparency and accountability make data more easily available—in both print and electronic formats—on insurance options, costs and eligibility, as well as provider quality and accountability. Consumers can be more involved as purchasers now, and they have "financial skin in the game." Given that 25 percent of health consumers have deductibles of $1,000 or more, they now have a greater financial interest in accessing this information. And more consumers are willing to go shopping for what they perceive as value. In a 2013 HealthPocket/Accenture online survey, reported by The Commonwealth Fund, 34 percent of health consumers surveyed would switch insurers to save on premium costs.[4,5,6]

Data Liberation and Transparency

Supported by vastly expanded computing capacity, the Health Data Initiative movement established within the U.S. Department of Health and Human Services (HHS), opened access to information on provider behavior related to safety and quality. As a result of this "democratization" of Internet-based health information, more people can analyze large data themselves, using previously unavailable information. Beyond data, the Internet's social media platforms enable peer-to-peer information sharing, connections to people with problems similar to their own, and the potential for cohesion around policy goals and advocacy.

Technology

Powerful microtechnology innovations are rapidly evolving, placing diagnostic and health information directly into the hands of consumers, often through smartphone apps and wearable devices such as activity trackers (Figure 1).

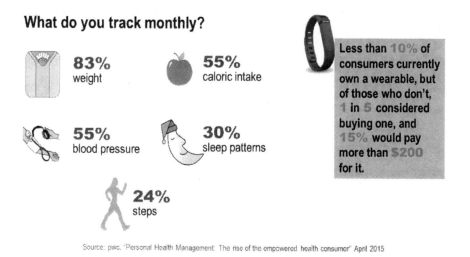

Figure 1. Consumers track health and fitness with technology.

New Attention to Consumer Experience and Attitudes

The Hospital Consumer Assessment of Healthcare Providers and Systems (HCAHPS) survey is the first national, standardized, publicly reported survey of patient experience. HCAHPS and the Patient Activation Measure (PAM), which assesses patient knowledge, skill and confidence for self-managing health, are supported by significant rewards (or penalties) in Medicare reimbursement rates based on the survey results (Figure 2).

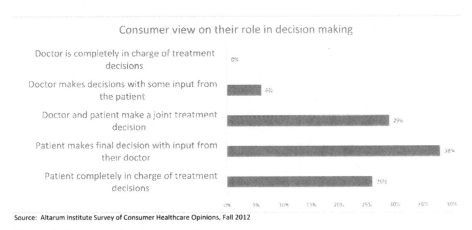

Source: Altarum Institute Survey of Consumer Healthcare Opinions, Fall 2012

Figure 2. Consumer healthcare opinions

Physician Self-Reforms

Some physician specialty associations are engaged in identifying overtreatment abuses, highlighting practices that lack evidence and could even provide potential harm. This initiative, under the banner of the Choosing Wisely campaign of the American Board of Internal Medicine (ABIM) and Consumer Reports, helps consumers and providers make better healthcare decisions. To spark meaningful conversations, leading specialty societies have created lists of "Five Things Physicians and Patients Should Question." Consumer Reports is developing and disseminating materials for patients to engage in their own consumer groups. A growing library of education modules and video resources also informs consumers.

The Changing Nature of Consumerism

The past decades have witnessed a "flattening of expert hierarchies." People are less likely to trust expert opinion. The "doc as god" syndrome has been replaced by a rise in skepticism. Advocacy movements like "nothing about me without me" call for the creation of "participatory medicine." More recently, The Pew Research Center Millennials studies document a widespread distrust of medical establishment practices and of the financial motives behind various treatment recommendations.[7]

In 1995, Kathy Giusti was diagnosed with multiple myeloma, a blood cancer considered incurable. She was a young mother, with a Harvard University master's degree and had been an executive at a pharmaceutical company. With a narrow window of time (under five years) to incite the drug discoveries that could save her, she quickly raised more than $450,000 from friends and launched a new organization, the Multiple Myeloma Research Foundation (MMRF). It operates under different rules than the traditionally more slow-moving disease associations: Applicant researchers must meet rapid and strict deadlines, be transparent in their progress and share preliminary findings with other potentially competitive researchers. The funding built an ad hoc collaborative of scientists who would accelerate the experimental process of drug discovery from clinical trials to commercialization of life-saving drugs. Dozens of new compounds have been tested and enough have proven worthy to ensure that Kathy would live. She is now a healthy mother, with a foundation that has raised hundreds of millions of dollars; and she has forever changed the course of multiple myeloma.[8]

What Are the Evolving Models of Patient Activation?

The Institute of Medicine's Quality of Healthcare in America project's publication, "Crossing the Quality Chasm: A New Health System for the 21st Century," envisions a care system "that is respectful of and responsive to individual patient preferences, needs and values, ensuring that patient values guide all clinical decisions."[9]

The following are some examples of the range of models that have been implemented on the road to patient activation:

- **Informed consent:** A well-intentioned process for getting permission before conducting a healthcare intervention on a person for treatment or research, informed consent is a reflection of the ethical principle of self-determination. Informed consent assumes a clear appreciation and understanding of the facts, implications and consequences of an action. However, informed consent has become a legal formality, often associated with long, difficult-to-understand forms with generalized information, providing little help to patients to explore their options or understand their risks.

- **Shared decision-making (SDM):** A collaborative process that allows patients and their providers to make healthcare decisions together takes into account the best scientific evidence available, as well as the patient's values and preferences. In SDM, patients receive information about various treatment options in an unbiased, balanced way so they can make an informed choice.

- **Evidence-based co-design:** This approach to improving patient experience and services, designed for the United Kingdom's National Health Service by The King's Fund, involves gathering experiences from patients and staff through in-depth interviewing, observations and group discussions, identifying key "touch points" (emotionally significant points) and assigning positive or negative feelings to them. They then create a short film from the patient interviews conveying how patients experience the service and show it to staff and patients.[10]

- **PatientsLikeMe:** According to their website,[11] this Web-based data-sharing platform was co-founded in 2004 by three Massachusetts Institute of Technology (MIT) engineers, including Benjamin and James Heywood, whose brother was diagnosed with ALS (Lou Gehrig's disease) at the age of 29. Today, PatientsLikeMe has four core values: putting patients in control, promoting transparency, fostering the sharing of discovery and breakthroughs, and creating virtual support—or what they call "wow".

Does Patient Activation Make a Measurable Difference?

According to the February 2013 issue of Health Affairs, there's emerging and growing evidence that care/outcomes are better with activated patients. The literature indicates that patients who are able to 1) self-manage symptoms/ problems; 2) engage in activities that maintain functioning and reduce health declines; 3) be involved in treatment and diagnostic choices; 4) collaborate with providers; 5) select providers and provider organizations based on performance or quality; and 6) navigate the healthcare system are likely to have better health outcomes and often at lower costs.[12]

Matt Might, a computer programmer trained at MIT, used his formidable knowledge of the Internet, as well as his international prominence as a blogger, to save his son's life and form a global network of parents of children with a rare genetic disorder known as NGLY1, which can cause developmental delays and liver disease. He knew that he had no time to spare in finding other children who might share his son's disease and form an advocacy group to accelerate recognition, research and treatment discovery. Finding sufferers of NGLY1 was like finding a needle in a haystack, and Matt knew he had to go global. He unleashed a "Google dragnet" (as described by writer Seth Mnookin) under the heading "Hunting Down My Son's Killer." The viral nature of his blog posting worked its magic, and parents began to surface from Turkey to Canada, Germany and the United Kingdom. These parent advocates also promoted research collaborations and, with the intervention of the National Institutes of Health (NIH), they made much progress. This is ample tribute to the power of the Internet to form global collaboratives among patients and researchers with a similar mission.[13]

In a TEDMED talk, "It's Time to Redesign Medical Data," Thomas Goetz offered six questions that every patient should ask his or her healthcare provider to create a feedback loop: Can I have my results? What does this mean? What are my options? What choices are now on the table? What's next? How do I integrate this information into the longer course of my life? The role of the healthcare provider as a partner is crucial to helping patients and their families answer these fundamental questions.

There's a tremendous amount of data now available to help people understand and manage their health issues. A greater challenge now is to find the information "needle" within the data haystack. It's reasonable to suggest that medical practices and health systems consider providing specially trained "informed navigators" to assist the activated patient to find useful credible sources. Some physicians are even forming their own patient support groups.

What Does Patient Activation Look Like to Providers?

Dr. Todd Wolynn is a pediatrician with a large multi-site practice. At each of his locations, he has a large, comfortable meeting room so that his patients can join in a host of peer support groups on topics as broad as expectant patient orientation, mom and baby yoga, prenatal breastfeeding, and sleep. On a

sunny winter morning, the meeting room in his Squirrel Hill office in Pittsburgh
was packed with young mothers of infants talking about breastfeeding. The
mothers learn childrearing skills and tips from each other while building
circles of friendship that could last well into their babies' teenage years.

In 1999, in conjunction with the American Board of Medical Specialties, the
Accreditation Council for Graduate Medical Education (ACGME), which approves all
medical residency programs in the United States, established six core competencies
that all resident physician must demonstrate before practicing medicine independently.
The core competencies include practice-based learning and improvement
(the ability to investigate and evaluate care of patients, appraise and assimilate
scientific evidence, and continuously improve patient care based on constant self-
evaluation and lifelong learning) and interpersonal and communication skills.

With the Internet, new apps and the "data liberation" movement leveling
the asymmetry of information between patients and health providers, health and
medical education is not keeping up and preparing young medical and practicing
health professionals to work in this new "information laden" environment. Many
consumers can now use their own computers or smartphones to instantaneously
discover updated information about their medical conditions (including their own
health records), recent research findings, new clinical trials, risks and appropriate
use of prescribed pharmaceuticals, plusses and minuses of surgical interventions,
and evidence confirming potential diagnostics.

To address this issue, the Jewish Healthcare Foundation (JHF) constructed
four fellowships (serving as collaboratives) aimed at graduate students, as well as
a series of "Champions" programs that challenge experienced professionals to re-
envision and virtually reinvent delivery systems, payment methods, information
technologies, and policies that define the patient experience and knowledge
base. These fellowships cover patient safety, quality improvement and information
technology, end of life, and the Salk fellowship, which investigates "disruptive"
health reforms beyond incremental changes). All four fellowships have a large
applicant pool and typically engage 25–40 students from multiple universities

and multiple professions over several months. Each year, the Champions programs engage a separate cohort of professionals including nurses, physicians, health administrators, business and public health leaders, occupational and physical therapists, pharmacists, medical assistants, emergency medical service workers, long-term care and certified nursing assistants, and now community health workers from multiple systems and practices in collaboratives for a year-long program of study, experimentation and skill development.

Case Study: The Hoy Family Story

By Libby Hoy

"I'm sorry Mrs. Hoy, I wish I had better news for you, but we don't expect your son to make it through the night." Those were the words that catapulted our family into the healthcare environment and thrust clinicians, therapists, social workers and pharmacists into our tiny family unit.

The next 23 years have been filled with 29 surgeries, countless physical and speech therapies, inpatient visits, outpatient visits and too many procedures to count. Getting a foothold in this environment was like drinking from a fire hose; we quickly learned the value of participating actively in our three sons' care. We were building Team Hoy, the clinical and support team we would need to help us care for the boys.

To be a team member meant clinicians had to integrate our priorities, values and goals into each decision. Our team supported our need for knowledge, providing access to medical records and guiding our search for the right diagnosis, which came seven years later. When things went awry, we worked together with the team to co-design solutions. This partnership approach empowered the boys to develop into young men who see their mitochondrial disease as a part of who they are, but certainly not the most important part. The value of that cannot be underestimated.

When the boys were young, we were at the hospital four to five times a week, when they weren't hospitalized. Imagine all the observations I made across the organization. From multiple inpatient units to the therapy centers, diagnostic areas, outpatient clinics, we were in the environment, acutely aware there were opportunities for improvement. Not only improvement for patients and families, but for staff and clinicians as well. Through the respectful partnerships we had developed in our clinical teams, we began to share our observations. Thus began my role of patient family advisor.

When I became the chair of the Miller Children's Parent Advisory Board, my peers and I could authentically inform improvement efforts. For instance, I had the opportunity to participate in a lean improvement effort to shorten wait times in one of the outpatient clinics where my sons received care. One of the physicians and I discussed the motivations (or lack thereof) of parents and clinicians to respond to one another. We expressed several negative assumptions until realizing the reason for the lack of response was that the phone tree was directing parents' calls to two lines of staff who were no longer with the organization; therefore no one was checking those message boxes. Without both of us in the room, that discovery would not have been made. As a result, we resolved the problem in 10 minutes at minimal cost.

Through these experiences, I began to see myself as a valuable resource to improvement efforts. It was obvious: The key is co-design of systems of care. The one perspective that crosses all silos of care is the patient and family, so it makes sense that their perspectives be included. This way, centering care on the patient and family not only provides a path to better outcomes, it becomes a functional construct for care delivery.

What Are Some Tools and Resources for Collaboratives?

There is a growing list of tools and resources that can be considered by collaboratives focused on patient engagement and activation. For example, to promote stronger engagement, Agency for Healthcare Research and Quality (AHRQ) developed "Guide to Patient and Family Engagement in Hospital Quality and Safety" to help patients, families and health professionals work together as partners to promote improvements in care. The guide focuses on the following strategies:

- Encourage patients and family members to participate as advisors.
- Promote better communication among patients, family members and healthcare professionals from the point of admission.
- Implement safe continuity of care by keeping the patient and family informed through nurse bedside change-of-shift reports.

Patient Activation Measure, as mentioned previously, is a tool developed by Judith Hibbard, Jean Stockard, Eldon R. Mahoney and Martin Tusler that assesses an individual's knowledge, skill and confidence for managing his or her own health and healthcare. Each activation level reveals insight into an array of health-related characteristics, including attitudes, motivators and outcomes. PAM is currently used in multiple countries.

Websites like PatientsLikeMe and Choosing Wisely, as previously mentioned, provide valuable information for patients and providers alike to consider options that suit their particular circumstances. As information resources and technology evolve over the next decade, collaboratives can play an important role in building on the democratization of information by guiding people to the best of what is available and helping them make informed healthcare decisions.

What Are Some New Models of Community, Patient and Provider Partnership?

There are many opportunities to develop new curricula, training and outreach vehicles targeted at empowering consumers. Collaboratives should take a lead in updating current practices to accommodate activated consumers. New models of patient communication start with good listening.

Motivational interviewing (MI) is a conversation style in which healthcare professionals and patients work together to discover the patient's own reasons to make positive behavioral changes and strengthen their commitment to change. Healthcare professionals and patients are treated as equal partners, each possessing useful knowledge that can help align the patient's actions with their stated life goals and values.

MI is being used successfully in a number of collaboratives throughout Pennsylvania. In each collaborative, outcomes indicate that when a practitioner places the goals of the patient at the center of the work, the outcomes are more satisfying, lasting and impactful.

The Center for Health Information Activation: CHIA is an initiative sponsored by the Jewish Healthcare Foundation and its supporting organizations, the Pittsburgh Regional Health Initiative and Health Careers Futures. CHIA's overarching goal is to help healthcare consumers and providers engage in meaningful, goal-directed collaboration and partnerships. CHIA began its work with a series of consumer "listening sessions." The results of those sessions are being used by the organization's boards, committees and partner organizations to develop strategies to support the engagement and activation of patients.

Collaboratives can take many forms. They don't have to last for months or years. Here's one example: More than 60 people gathered in the QIT Training Center of the Jewish Healthcare Foundation in July of 2015. They represented a mix of practitioners, association directors, researchers, health advocates, attorneys, educators and the public sector. What they had in common was a willingness to respect and activate health consumers. The unusual gathering was intended to spark a regional movement of health activation. After examining common elements of successful health reform movements of the past 50 years, the participants broke into teams and entered a competition for the best designed strategy to activate consumers around six critical health problems. In effect, they applied MI techniques to collective behavioral change.

What Are Some Topics for Regional Interdisciplinary Learning and Action Collaboratives?

Some current topics lend themselves well to collective conversation, learning and action.

Once considered a topic to be avoided, end-of-life care fails many families and patients and could be vastly improved. This topic covers intriguing medical ethical and philosophical issues and lends itself to collective examination. "Closure," a unique educational model developed by JHF, was designed as a learning, community-organizing and planning forum built around six structured community conversations. Columnist Ellen Goodman, Institute for Healthcare Improvement and writer Dr. Atul Gawande are generating much interest in this topic, and many communities throughout the United States are using the Closure model.

Women are excellent ambassadors for health. Caring for themselves, their parents and children, they can build healthy living practices into family life. To further this, JHF convened Working Hearts, a community coalition of women's organizations that engaged natural networks of women across more than 40 organizations to identify and avoid heart disease as a milestone on the road to good health. The campaign, which lasted five years and reached

233

tens of thousands of women and providers, created a range of educational materials and engagement opportunities. Now many health insurers and the American Heart Association have picked up the mantle and engaged women in heart health and so much more.

How Can Collaboratives Reach the Media?

Training, community education, and activation of the public and providers need not just occur through traditional means. Collaboratives can create and distribute original communication resources through a variety of communication vehicles (television, online and written anthologies) for community members and providers.

For the past 20-plus years, JHF has had an ongoing strategy of partnership with its local public television station, WQED, creating a unique learning and engagement opportunity. In 2012, WQED aired a JHF-produced documentary, "The Last Chapter," which explores six individuals (ranging in age from a few months to more than 90) with life-threatening illnesses and their families, and their respective decisions for how they handled their illnesses and prepared for their deaths. The award-winning 60-minute film was picked up for national distribution by Public Broadcasting Service (PBS) in more than 200 cities. It's available online as well, and is accompanied by a discussion guide aimed at triggering conversations, learning, and action by collaboratives and communities.

In 2014, WQED aired a documentary funded by JHF and the Josiah Macy Foundation, "The Empowered Patient." This half-hour special looks at the new role of patients and healthcare providers in a world where information is more readily available than ever before. With patients doing more of their own research and connecting with other patients online, healthcare providers are often interacting with more engaged, informed and empowered patients. The documentary explores these changing relationships.

Over the course of the past nine years, Creative Nonfiction Foundation has completed five healthcare anthologies written by providers and families around such diverse topics as error, patient safety, end of life and mental illness. Collectively these anthologies allow readers to hear firsthand narratives of the healthcare system—the good, the bad and the ugly. This form of nonfiction engages providers, patients and families, allowing them to "see themselves" through stories. First-person narratives have proven to be very powerful, as evidenced by the popularity of Atul Gawande's book, "Being Mortal," which has served as a great conversation starter among communities, patients and providers.

Conclusion

Collaboratives must embrace the "new patient" profile—the increasingly activated and informed patient who is in charge of his or her health and healthcare decisions. The activated patient will demand new relationships with medical professionals and facilities. That new relationship is relatively unexplored and developed, particularly among practitioners and health profession schools. In this model, the medical professional is a partner and supporter rather than an omniscient decision-maker, and the patients are no longer supplicants asking for information about themselves, their health or any particular condition.

Collaboratives among researchers, clinicians, consumers, purchasers and payers are a vital resource in this new alignment. There is a strategic imperative to embrace the new profile, and collaboratives in particular should advance new attitudes toward, and practices with, patients and families by their own composition and way of doing business. Collective behavior change through collaboratives based on the principles of successful health and social movements of the past could ride the wave of an increasingly active consumer base.

[1] Conway, J., Nathan, D., Benz, E., Shulman, L., Sallan, S., & Ponte, P. (June 2-6 2006). Key learning from the Dana-Farber Cancer Institute's 10-year patient safety journey. *American Society of Clinical Oncology 2006 Educational Book, 42nd Annual Meeting*, (pp. 615-619). Atlanta, GA.

[2] Ponte, P., Conlin, G., Conway, J., Grant, S., Medeiros, C., Nies, J., et al. (2003). Making patient-centered care come alive: Achieving full integration of the patient's perspective. *Journal of Nursing Administration* , 33 (2), 82-90.

[3] *Pew Research Center*. Retrieved from Millennials: www.pewresearch.org/topics/millennials

[4] *HealthPocket*. (n.d.). Retrieved from Online Survey: https://www.healthpocket.com/healthcare-research/surveys#.VgK4rWRViko

[5] *Accenture Report*. (2013, Sept 16). Retrieved from U.S. Research Findings Consumer Health Survey: https://www.accenture.com/us-en/insight-accenture-consumer-survey-patient-engagement-summary.aspx

[6] *The Commonwealth Fund*. (2013, April). Retrieved from http://www.commonwealthfund.org/

[7] *Pew Research Center*. Retrieved from Millennials: www.pewresearch.org/topics/millennials

[8] Groopman, J. (2008, Jan 28). Buying a Cure: What business know-how can do for disease. *The New Yorker, Medical Dispatch* .

[9] Institute of Medicine. (2001). *Crossing the Quality Chasm: A New Health System for the 21st Century.* Washington DC: National Academy Press. Pg 3.

[10] Boyd, H., McKernon, S., Mullin, B., & Old, A. (2012). *Auckland District Health Board* (ISSN: 1175-8716 ed., Vol. 125). Auckland, New Zealand: Med J.

[11] *Patients Like Me*. Retrieved from https://www.patientslikeme.com/

[12] Greene, J., Hibbard, J., Sacks, R., & al., e. (2013). When Seeing the Same Physician, Highly Activated Patients Have Better Care Experiences Than Less Activated Patients. *Health Affairs* , 32 (7), 1295-1305.

[13] Mnookin, S. (2014, July 21). One of a Kind, What do you do if your child has a condition that is new to science? *The New Yorker, Medical Dispatch*.

CHAPTER 13

Communication for Collaboratives

By Andrew Cooper, Jenny Kowalczuk, and Alan Willson, Ph.D.
Communication Strategies—Project JOINTS by Jo Ann Endo, MSW
Using Stories to Inspire Change by Virginia McBride RN, MPH

Introduction

Quality improvement is a team sport—you can't do it alone. In addition to developing methods and measures, delivering training and offering advice, improvement leaders must inspire, motivate, persuade and engage all kinds of people at all levels. The task is significant—demanding that we apply both technical and soft skills to succeed. We know that 25 percent or more improvement projects fail, but we're just beginning to ask why.[1]

In a study that examined the reasons for success and failure in improvement projects in a hospital, researchers found that leadership was closely related to both success and failure[2] in quality improvement; others have found the absence of effective, strategic communications may be another root cause. We all know about great improvement work that failed because it relied on one person's efforts and wasn't widely adopted. Failed projects represent missed opportunities for patients as well as wasted healthcare services talent and resources.

Effective communication that supports greater efficiency for healthcare services and better outcomes for patients doesn't "just happen." For communication to be effective it requires fact-finding, planning and systematic implementation—much like setting up a multi-center collaborative or designing an improvement project. This chapter will help you develop an integrated communication strategy to help you meet quality-improvement goals.

Is This Chapter for You?

This chapter is for anyone responsible for delivering quality improvement. It will help if you're delivering communications on your own or as a team, or if you're hiring a communications expert. It's written for use by improvement teams, but if you're working with a communications expert, it will give you an essential understanding of how communication strategy is built, what to watch for and how to get the best from your communications team.

Whatever your background, experience and role in quality improvement, you don't need previous experience or skill in strategic communications to apply the framework we're sharing.

We developed the framework after delivering communications for a successful national campaign.[3] It includes six steps to plan strategic communication and integrate it into your collaborative, project or campaign. The steps are based on evidence and experience from the fields of communications and public relations. Following are the steps:

1. **Aim:** What do you want to achieve?
2. **Audience:** Who do you need to engage?
3. **Message:** What do you need to say?
4. **Channels:** How will you reach your audience?

5. **Story:** How will you engage your audience?
6. **Review:** What was the impact and what will you learn for next time?

The 1000 Lives Campaign

We're introducing the strategic communication framework in this chapter based on our experience delivering the 1000 Lives Campaign in Wales. We launched the two-year campaign in 2008 to improve patient safety and increase quality of care across the National Health Service in Wales.[4] Based on the Institute for Healthcare Improvement's 100,000 Lives Campaign, the 1000 Lives Campaign aimed to save an additional 1,000 lives and prevent 50,000 episodes of harm during the two years of the campaign.

Our communication strategy enabled us to build momentum to keep the focus on campaign goals during the two-year period, support local organizations and work effectively at scale. Just as technical skills deliver improvement, the discipline of communication to support collaboratives can play a major part in saving lives, improving outcomes and motivating and rewarding staff.

The 1000 Lives Campaign was firmly rooted in improvement methodology and applied a collaborative approach across six clinical settings. Key aspects of the campaign included:

- The goal to facilitate, not direct, improvement.
- An absence of regional or local targets; teams and organizations across our health service set their own priorities.
- Voluntary participation at all levels, from boardroom to bedside.
- Frontline healthcare staff as the key audience.

Strategic Communication

In the complex healthcare environment, "communication" means different things to different people and in some cases may lack substance. This discussion of communication focuses on embedding strategic communication into collaborative work to support participation and accelerate adoption across processes and systems.

Effective strategic communication supports participation, maintains momentum toward quality-improvement goals, and gives compelling reasons for participation at the front line and support in the boardroom. It supports behavior change and facilitates change in organizations and their cultures. Strategic communication is part of the discipline of public relations; it's planned and uses evidence to inform decision-making. We can define it as...

"...the intentional communication undertaken by a business or non-profit organization, sometimes by a less well-structured group. It has a purpose and a plan, in which alternatives are considered and decisions are justified. Invariably, strategic communication is based on research and subject to eventual evaluation." [5]

Strategic communication is intentional because it's thoughtfully designed and planned to support a larger goal. Its purpose is clearly defined and measurable, and there's a plan that uses evidence to identify *what* will be communicated, *who* will be reached and *how* they will be reached. When delivered, strategic communication reviews activity to find out what worked and what didn't, so more effective communication can be delivered in the future.

Using strategic communication in quality-improvement work doesn't just offer more effective ways of delivering instructions; it presents greater opportunities for reflection, invites action and nurtures relationships on which effective collaboration can be built. Strategic communication is about relationship building, and it demands we shift our focus from broadcasting and instructing to collaborating and motivating.

We hope the strategic approach to communication that we present here will encourage stronger, more constructive relationships among leaders of improvement projects, campaigns, collaboratives and initiatives, and the healthcare staff they want to involve and inspire.

What You Need to Succeed

The next section of this chapter describes in detail the six steps we developed while delivering the 1000 Lives Campaign. You don't need prior knowledge or skills in communication; simply follow the steps to develop a strategy aligned with your quality-improvement goals. The steps are simple, but they're not easy. You'll need to involve others to think through the questions, gather information and consider tactics. Implemented with dedication, the framework will help you succeed.

The Communication Framework

There are six core components to our communication framework. Each component is essential and, like frameworks used to achieve improved patient outcomes, each component builds on the next. The six steps— aim, audience, message, channels, story and review—are explored in detail, with practical examples from our experience during the 1000 Lives Campaign in Wales.

1. Aim: What do you want to achieve?
Communication must align with the goals of your quality-improvement work. This means getting involved in the planning process when the overall goals are being determined. The larger collaborative goals must inform your supporting

communication goals. If communication is on the agenda at the beginning of the planning process, it will naturally become integral to the project.

The communication role during the planning stage is to ensure goals are clear, concise and easy to articulate. If you can't say it, you can't share it. Communications can help tighten poorly focused or worded goals to strengthen and clarify them. Think of NASA's aim of "putting a man on the moon" and the complexity that simple goal embodies. Aspire to develop goals that are SMART: Specific, Measureable, Achievable, Relevant and Time-based.

When you've aligned communications with your larger goals, then:

- Messages will be clear and focused.
- The stories you use to communicate your goals will be more relevant and compelling.
- You'll more effectively communicate common goals.
- People will collaborate to meet the goals.
- It will be easier to measure progress.

The 1000 Lives Campaign aimed to save an additional 1,000 lives in Welsh healthcare over a two-year span, and the communication plan was measured against this goal. Focusing on the overall goal, we set communication goals to support it. These included the:

- Number of organizations that would take part in the campaign.
- Number of staff attending learning and training days.
- Commitment of teams to deliver interventions.
- Commitment of teams and organizations to measure success.

We developed a strategy aligned with the campaign goal so that our communication activity had purpose and drive. We knew that to save 1,000 additional lives we would need to engage frontline healthcare workers in the campaign and win their support. We were constantly communicating, explaining and celebrating successes to maintain momentum toward goals.

When you set a goal, make it easy to understand: Use numbers instead of proportions. Numbers—like saved lives, fewer bed days and prevented infections—are motivating and give people something tangible to work toward. Counting is a very simple act and it's engaging, meaningful and transparent. Proportions and other statistics, on the other hand, may be confusing. For example, reducing pressure ulcers by 20 percent is hard to assess and may inspire confusion or questions: How many people did this affect? Does it make a difference in my department? Is this someone else's project or concern?

Be very clear about what you want to achieve, and don't let your goals or outcomes be side-tracked by proxy (or process) measures. For example, a hydration campaign may use the proxy measure of a patient's fluid intake to measure progress, but the goal should be to reduce the risk of urinary tract infections and other complications—not to increase fluid intake. Increasing fluid intake is just a tactic in a larger strategy.

It can also help to think of overall goals in terms of the people they impact. For example:

- What do you want people to do? In the 1000 Lives Campaign we wanted frontline staff to sign up and take part in the campaign.
- What do you want to make happen? In our campaign, we ultimately wanted to reduce avoidable deaths.

Broad, general goals usually lead to disappointment. Clear, defined, measurable and achievable goals lead to success. Take your time to get the goals right. Frame them positively if you can—save lives, don't reduce mortality. Use expert help if needed, from senior management to those handling and analysing relevant data. Experts can help you focus on areas where your work will have measurable impact. Resist the temptation to set goals quickly and move on to implementation issues—these are often easy to deal with, while getting the goals right may not be.

Alignment

Our communication strategy was closely aligned with the overall campaign goals and developed around two points of focus:

- To admit the problem—without sensationalizing or over-promising.
- To make participation voluntary for organizations, individuals and teams— which was enabling for healthcare staff in the pressured environment of our national health services.

Early on in planning, we recognized a number of communication challenges:

- Clinical staff felt their desire to deliver safe, quality care was frustrated by "the system," and some didn't believe such a high level of harm existed or was avoidable.
- Admitting to the problem of safety, the campaign ran the risk of reducing confidence in health services.
- "Target fatigue" among healthcare staff could make buy-in for a new campaign hard to achieve.

Without tackling these challenges, any one of them could have derailed the campaign. We addressed the issues by speaking directly to staff concerns, calling on their vocation and professionalism and desire to make a difference to others, to win their active participation in the work needed to reach our goals. By affirming vocation and professionalism, we made a direct appeal to the hearts and minds of frontline healthcare staff and set a warm, human tone for all our communications.

If you can bring communications into early planning for your collaborative, you'll develop a strategy strongly aligned with overall goals. When you do this, your improvement work and communication have the best possible chance of success.

2. Audience: Who do you need to engage?

A successful collaborative requires reaching out to different groups of people—your audiences. The more sharply you define and understand your audiences, the easier it will be to reach them and deliver your messages.

You'll have several audiences, but you should prioritize them based on who most influences your success or failure. The temptation is to put something out there "for everyone" and hope it works—which we like to call the "spray-and-pray" approach. With sufficient planning, you'll be able to tease out distinct groups and their needs and preferences, then design targeted communications that speak directly to them.

To help distinguish among audiences, ask these questions:

- Among the senior manager teams, which are critical to the project's success? Which high-level meetings could we use to communicate our message(s)?
- Do we need to focus on clinical specialties or cut across specialties?
- Are there professional bodies whose support would strengthen our work?
- Who has interest in the outcomes of our work, inside and outside our organization?
- Which patients will need to support the project?
- Does the public have an interest?

At this point, you may want to do some stakeholder research. This doesn't have to be complicated, expensive or time-consuming. Schedule five- or 10-minute phone calls with someone from each audience.

Ask how they see your work, what they think could stop the work from succeeding, and why they may or may not get involved. Find out about information-sharing opportunities with groups; these may include professional networks, meetings, events or regular briefings.

Use what you discover to sketch short profiles of your audiences: their motivations, needs, concerns and priorities; their regular meetings and information-sharing channels; and their likely level of engagement with your collaborative work. Remember that audiences aren't homogeneous; they're made up of individuals. So think of a typical person in each audience and how, when and why you would speak to them. This will allow you to reach them directly with relevant, useful communication. With a sense of what makes your audience tick, you'll be able to deliver messages that speak to their interests, through channels they find most accessible.

You'll probably discover many groups needing targeted communications, so unless you have unlimited resources, you'll have to prioritize. It's always better to focus on a small number of audiences and deliver the right messages, in the right format and through the right channels, than to work poorly with a large number of audiences.

Our communication strategy for the 1000 Lives Campaign had to cut across specialties and roles and be appropriate for all levels of seniority, so we kept our audience categories broad. We identified six audiences, including:

1. People who will lead the campaign nationally—or local campaign leads.
2. People who will deliver the campaign—e.g., frontline healthcare staff.
3. People who will provide direct support for campaign delivery—e.g., staff from the Government Department of Health and Social Care, local health board managers and local communication officers.

4. People who will support the campaign and influence the public—
    e.g., politicians, academics, advocacy groups and the media.
5. People with an interest but not a role in the campaign—e.g., staff
    from voluntary organizations and health legal experts.
6. Patients and the public—e.g., patients, families and friends of
    patients, and the wider public.

Our priority audience were the people who would ultimately make the
campaign happen: the frontline healthcare staff. Identifying this primary
audience unlocked the entire strategy and our messages, channels, images
and content then fell into place. We knew we needed to maintain the rock-
solid support from the high-level political and executive leadership. But we
knew that if we didn't have results, we didn't have a campaign. And this
made our frontline staff our number one priority and informed much of our
communication work.

3. Message: What do you need to say?

Your messages are the lifeblood of your strategy, so they need to be the right
ones. They must link your goals with actions. Your messages need to be clear,
but you don't have to deliver award-winning advertising copy. Instead, drill
down to the essential information needed to deliver the outcomes you want.
You should have a small number of core messages and these can each be
adapted for your different audiences. Your core messages must inform all
of your communications materials and be delivered consistently, over and
over, in different ways and through different channels. Consistency in your
messaging is the key to success—so be sure to get your messages right.

When you've done the work to understand what motivates your audiences,
crafting messages for your audiences should become easier. Write messages
in the language the audience uses. For example, reducing "hospital-acquired
thrombosis" is appropriate if your audience is medical staff, but if it's patients

or the public you need to reach, you may want to use "clots" as that's the language your audience understands.

Effective messages call on emotions to engage and inspire action. Give all of your messages an emotional driver like "saving lives" or "the best outcome for every patient every time." This is as important for messages targeted to your chief executive as those for your nursing staff. Aim to motivate and inspire, looking for a positive way to frame your messages. Keeping messages consistent and positive, even when dealing with challenging areas of practice and different target groups, address fears and concerns and can be reassuring.

The language you use will have a massive impact, so think carefully about your choice of words. Be direct and personal; speak to your audiences' emotions and aspirations as if you were in conversation with them.

In our campaign, even though we aimed to save 1,000 additional lives and prevent 50,0000 episodes of unnecessary harm, our key message didn't mention death or harm at all:

"NHS Wales staff save lives every day. The 1000 Lives Campaign will help them save even more."

This message positioned the campaign positively, as something building on good work, instead of being another top-down initiative to knock staff on what they *weren't* doing. It tapped into the reason why many people went into healthcare in the first place: to make a difference. The time we spent on getting this message right proved crucial to the success of the campaign. It became the language used by everyone and quickly and consistently set the tone for the campaign ethos and aspirations.

Take Your Time

With so much to consider, it's important not to rush the messaging. Give yourself enough time to share ideas with colleagues, draft and redraft messages, and find out how they're received by your target audiences. When you test your messages, be sure to involve the people your message will impact, whether they are frontline healthcare staff or chief executives and directors. You don't need to run big, expensive focus groups—it can be just as effective to work informally by sounding your messages out on one or two people to begin with and a small group when they're being finalized.

4. Channels: How will you reach your audience?

This step builds directly on the work you've done to identify audiences and which ones need to be the main priority. When you start to look at the channels available for delivering your message, you'll bring what you've learned about your audiences. This will allow you to make informed choices instead of guesses about which channels to use. If you've done a good job and know your audiences well, the channels for reaching them should be clear.

Digital channels offer the possibility of low-cost, high-quality, and instantaneous publication. While this is great news, the downside is that communications must now cut through a massive amount of noise. It pays to choose a few channels wisely, and invest more time and effort in each one to gain maximum impact. The most effective channels may be the ones you could easily overlook, such as workplace notice boards or influential people.

People As Channels

In all organizations there are people with the power to influence others. These influencers can, if you win their support, become significant channels for your work. We established a faculty of quality improvement experts drawn from all disciplines. They supported the campaign by forging partnerships with professional bodies, using their existing communication networks to promote our messages, and informally sharing information with their peers to promote campaign engagement.

There are influencers in your organization at all levels, with the potential to become advocates for your work, sharing your progress, affirming messages and maintaining momentum toward your goals. Finding and supporting these champions will give your work sustainable impetus, creating a "pull" for improvement activity.

Choose Your Channels Like You'd Choose a Team

Channels should complement each other in the same way that different roles come together to deliver complex surgical procedures in an operating room. This will allow you to deliver your message in different ways and repackage content produced for one channel to tell the story on another. Good content repackaging makes your messages come alive for different audiences through different channels.

Case Study: Ask About Clots—Repackaging Content for Different Audiences

In April 2014, 1000 Lives Improvement launched the Ask About Clots campaign. The campaign aimed to increase public awareness about the risk of developing a blood clot (thrombosis) while in the hospital. The campaign message was to encourage patients to ask about their personal risk of developing a clot while in the hospital so they could be assessed and treated appropriately. A wide variety of content was created to share key messages and increase engagement:

- **Website (microsite):** This acted as a hub for content and resources; it was accessible to the public as well as health professionals and the media.
- **Case studies:** These supported internal communications and were for media use.
- **Blogs:** We built awareness and understanding with healthcare staff by publishing blogs by thought leaders.
- **Videos:** These included an animated information video for use in healthcare waiting rooms, and a news-style video that included a clip with the clinical lead and a case study.

- **Social Media:** We worked with a social media agency to craft engaging, shareable content with relevant hashtags.
- **Infographic:** This reinforced key messages in an accessible format for print and social media.

In addition, we produced communication packs for internal teams to use, press packs, email newsletters and photos. We also organized a launch event, integrated our campaign with a larger UK campaign and syndicated news stories across the NHS in Wales.

Internal Channels

In the 1000 Lives Campaign, we invested in internal communication and developed channels unique to the campaign, including a website, email newsletter, print newsletters and a range of print media to support communication teams. We worked to build strong relationships with our faculty, medical directors, senior management groups and professional bodies. We also invested in generating content to keep channels active, staging many events and video interviews as the campaign progressed to deliver a range of communication to tell our story.

We thought of creative ways to keep bringing the campaign to everyone's attention, by staging events, celebrating small victories and marking milestones. All too often communication work is all launch and no follow through—depending on the scale of your work and the channels you use, you may want to make sure you refresh content daily, weekly or monthly. Social media channels like Twitter are more demanding, and to get the most from them you should post several times a day.

Deliver your messages as though you were running a political campaign. Keep the messages consistent and repeat them frequently. If you get consistent feedback that one or more of your messages isn't working, only then make a change: Messages take a long time to be recognized and trusted. If you're delivering improvement work over a long period of time, e.g., within a three-year multi-center collaborative, it's essential to maintain interest in the work and keep people engaged. Think of new ways to deliver content, tell stories about the work, mark successes and profile the people involved, but always keep your messaging consistent.

Case Study: Communication Strategies—Project JOINTS

Jo Ann Endo, MSW

The Institute for Healthcare Improvement (IHI) created the Project JOINTS initiative to increase the use of three evidence-based surgical site infection (SSI) reduction practices in hip and knee replacements in more than 200 hospitals in 10 U.S. states and Washington, D.C. IHI based the approach on what we learned from using the infrastructure developed during the 100,000 and 5 Million Lives Campaigns.

RAND published a study on Project JOINTS[6] (*BMJ Quality & Safety*) that found one of the strongest predictors of adoption of the SSI reduction practices was engagement of hospital leadership, physicians and frontline staff Enhancing hospital engagement was a primary focus of Project JOINTS communications.

Project JOINTS decided to support its communication strategy with an in-house communications specialist. Once the team identified its key communication goals, audiences, channels and story, it designed specific materials and messages to engage various stakeholders. The Project JOINTS team used a range of strategies, including:

Target Audience: Surgeons

- Handout designed for surgeons, summarizing evidence for the three interventions
- Videos, including interviews with a patient describing the consequences of an SSI, and a surgeon urging other surgeons to participate

Target Audience: Implementation Team

- How-to guide providing implementation advice for clinicians, patient educators, and others
- Team members speaking and sharing their experiences
- Webinars to present evidence, share best practices and teach quality improvement
- Electronic mailing list offering tools, resources, webinar materials and recordings; a place to ask questions and find peer-to-peer support

Target Audience: Patients and Consumers

- Education materials to help patients reduce their SSI risk

Target Audience: Leadership

- Documents describing the business case to promote leadership engagement
- Customizable press release template for organizations to announce their participation to local media

Target Audience: General/Multi-Audience

- Project JOINTS website for free access to tools and resources
- Media outreach resulting in a story in a major national publication

5. Story: How will you engage your audience?

"Those who tell the stories, rule the world."
—Plato

During the campaign, one care audit on an Intensive Therapy Unit picked up an issue that was having a large, negative impact on patients—noise from closing refuse bin lids.

A patient recovering from serious injuries complained, saying the slamming lids woke her when she was resting and the sharp sound made her feel angry. When staff investigated, they found the slamming bin lids caused the loudest spikes of sound on the ward and exceeded recommended World Health Organization noise levels for hospital wards. The noise from the bins was louder than telephones ringing, monitor alarms or staff talking between beds.

The bins were replaced with new ones that had a silent shutting mechanism. The difference was tangible not only to patients, who reported enjoying uninterrupted sleep, but to staff as well, who found it easier to concentrate with less interruption from noise.

For patients, safety and quality improvements can make the difference between illness and recovery, or even life and death. For staff, victories are hard won and deserve celebrating. Stories bring together the experience of quality-improvement work in human terms, showing how and why your goals will and must be achieved. Your messages give structure and focus to your communication, but stories create the narrative.

Stories are adaptable and can be shared with a wide range of audiences inside and outside the organization. They can help win support for your work at every level, from the CEO in the boardroom to the orderlies and porters.

Stories can be used for teaching, raising awareness and engaging staff at conferences and meetings. They reward success and keep everyone pushing hard for change. People remember them, share them and use them to shape their own choices and behavior.

Collecting stories needs a network of supporters at the frontline who can be your eyes and ears. Make it easy for them to share stories; give opportunities in newsletters and at events. Stories don't always need to be narrative: A video or single image can be just as powerful. Accept stories of all kinds; stories of success in care can be just as powerful as stories of failure.

Expect the Unexpected

Stories don't need to be complicated to be effective. They can come from the most unexpected places and be about the most unexpected improvements.

Stories like the one about the bins demonstrate to others that change is possible, that improvements that matter to patients aren't always complicated or difficult to achieve, and that improvement work is supported by managers willing to act on staff concerns. Develop an ear for good stories. They're often mentioned in passing and it's important to collect them—so record video, write them down or interview the people involved. Stories create understanding and build momentum to drive your initiative forward. This is especially important after the early quick wins when staff face the hard work of sustaining improvement.

Just as they don't always need to be complicated, they also don't need to be extraordinary or superlatives: You may risk alienating those whose equally vigorous efforts have come to nothing for reasons outside their control. Be even-handed, look for success of all kinds and noble failures, at all levels and among all kinds of people. "If they can do it, so can we" is the attitude you can help to promote. Always make sure your stories link directly to the overall collaborative or improvement work. Without a clear link to your goals, they have no strategic value.

6. Review: What was the impact, and what will you learn for next time?

When reviewing your communications work, systematically work through each of the five preceding steps in this framework:

1. Was the overall goal right, and how well did communications support it?
2. Were the right audiences selected? Were they too broad, too narrow or the wrong audiences?
3. Did the messages engage the audiences? Did the messages support the goals and were they clear and memorable?
4. Was the narrative of the work developed correctly—did it have any unintentional positive or detrimental consequences?
5. What were the most powerful stories with the biggest impact? What did you learn from collecting them, and would you do anything differently?

Reviewing your communications work as part of the evaluation process will show its impact on the overall quality-management effort. It may also reveal powerful tactics you can use again, or weaker areas of your strategy that you should strengthen before using for another project. Reviewing the strategy, what you delivered and what happened offers the opportunity to refine your future communications work.

Measures

Measurement is a key aspect of improvement methodology—and should be applied to your communications work. If you can't measure it, how will you know you're making a difference? How will you know how to improve? Measures must focus on outcomes, aligned to overall goals and not just activity. This is difficult, but it's possible.

Communication has traditionally relied on measuring output as media coverage; e.g., minutes of broadcast, column inches in newspapers or number of website visitors.

These measures are useful, especially to assess the effectiveness of external communication activity. But these measures alone don't give us much insight into the impact of our communications work. Comments on blogs and news items and shares through social media can tell us a lot about how people are engaging with a campaign. We can conduct more telephone interviews and focus groups to find out what people remember about the campaign and its key messages. We can capture and analyse web data to find out which pages were most viewed, what resources were downloaded and how long people stayed on our website as part of evaluating our work.

Conclusion

The communications framework we've presented was designed to make it easy for anyone working in quality improvement to produce a communication strategy to support their work. The framework is:

- **Easily scalable:** Use it small, use it big!
- **Not context-specific:** It can be used for any improvement project.

Using Stories to Inspire Change

By Virginia McBride RN, MPH

Alexa Kersting, a teenager suffering from interstitial lung disease, waited on the transplant list for a lung that never came. She died in 2004 at age 14.

The next year Alexa's mom, Monica, addressed an audience of hundreds of organ donor and transplant professionals, imploring them to remember her daughter. She reminded them that every lung is precious and no transplantable lung should ever be left behind.

The healthcare professionals who heard Monica's message that day were participating in a collaborative to increase organ donors and transplants in the U.S. They accepted "Alexa's Challenge" to increase available lungs and decrease waiting-list deaths.

Largely as a result of this call to action, the number of annual lung transplants increased from 1,405 in 2005 to 1,925 in 2014. The number of annual lung waiting-list deaths decreased from 373 to 216.

This is just one breath-taking example of how donors, recipients and their families inspire doctors and nurses to participate in the organ donation and transplant process.

- **Not skill-dependent:** It can be used by clinical staff, managers or anyone else, and will build communication across teams in your organization.
- **Collaborative:** It supports collaboration, enabling quality-improvement initiatives to integrate communication.
- **Empowering:** Working with communication teams is a new, important tool for quality-improvement and collaborative leaders.

The framework will make your communications even more effective when you use it:

- Step-by-step, as each step builds on the last.
- As an integral part of your collaborative and not in isolation.
- With your own context-specific measures.

We realized the importance of strategic communication to support collaboratives when we designed and ran the 1000 Lives Campaign.

For us, the benefits were described by one of our senior faculty advisors as being like "applying an exponential in math."[7]

The impact and sustainability of collaboratives were multiplied many times, and understanding of quality-improvement culture grew as people saw their work recognized, could share learning and understood their contribution toward campaign goals.

We believe there's a real case for building strategic communications into collaborative methodology—not as a bolt-on extra or nice-to-have, but as an essential component of a larger process.

Further Reading

Goals
Sustaining lean healthcare programmes: a practical survival guide; Mark Eaton and Simon Phillips, 2008, ecademy press, Penryn.

Audiences
Can I change your mind? The craft and art of persuasive writing, Lindsay Camp, 2007 A&C Black. See Chapter 3, Understanding your reader.
The Jelly Effect: how to make your communication stick, Andy Bounds, 2007, Capstone.

Messages
The invisible grail: how brands can use words to engage with audiences; John Simmons, Cyan 2006
Oglivy on Advertising, David Oglivy 1983 Prion.

Stories
The Power of Positive Deviance, Pascale, R, Sternin J, Sternin M, 2010, Harvard Business School Press.
The Heart of Change, Real life stories of how people change their organizations. John P Kotter and Dan Cohen, 2012, Harvard Business Review Press.

Channels

Randall S, 2015, Quick Guide: Using communication approaches to spread improvement. Health Foundation, http://www.health.org.uk/publications/using-communications-approaches-to-spread-improvement/

De Silva D, 2014, Evidence Scan, Spreading improvement ideas, tips from empirical research; Health Foundation, http://www.health.org.uk/publications/spreading-improvement-ideas/ Accessed 14 April 2015

Review

Evaluation your communications tools: what works, what doesn't? The Westminster Model; Westminster City Council, 2011, http://www3.westminster.gov.uk/Newdocstores/publications_store/communications/evaluating_your_comms_aw_lr-1319206316.pdf Accessed 4th May 2015

---

[1] Eaton, M., & Phillips, S. (2008). *Sustaining lean healthcare programmes - a practical survival guide.* Penryn, Cornwall: Ecademy Press.

[2] Creasy, T. (2014, October). Why do Improvement Projects Fail? *Hospital Review.*

[3] Cooper, A. (n.d.). From Exploring the role of communications in quality improvement: A case study of the 1000 Lives Campaign in NHS Wales.

[4] 1000 Lives Plus – The STOP campaign.

[5] Smith, R. D. (2009). *Strategic Planning for Public Relations* (3rd edition ed.). Routledge, London: Lawrence Erlbaum Associate, Inc., Publishers.

[6] Khodyakov, D., Ridgely, M., Huang, C., DeBartolo, K., Sorbero, M., & Schneider, E. (2015, Nov 5). Project JOINTS: What factors affect bundle adoption in a voluntary quality improvement campaign? *BMJ Qal Saf* .

[7] Willson, A. (2015, April 22). *Exploring the role of communications in quality improvement.* Retrieved May 4, 2015 from http://www.health.org.uk/blog/exploring-the-role-of-communications-quality-improvement/

CHAPTER 14

Evaluating Effectiveness and the Future of Collaboratives

By Bruce Spurlock, M.D.
The Champion Model: An Alternative Collaborative by
Karen Wolk Feinstein, Ph.D. and Susan Elster, Ph.D.

"Life begins at the end of your comfort zone."

– Neale Donald Walsch

Introduction

It was one of those ordinary mornings in the hospital several years ago. Rounding on my patients, I saw Mary, a long-known patient, admitted the previous evening for shortness of breath.

She greeted me with excitement. "Good morning, Dr. Spurlock. I'm feeling much better this morning."

What I saw on the hand-off note from the admitting physician was "elderly female CHF SOB." When I went to examine her, there it was—a new murmur.

Naturally, dozens of thoughts and diagnoses raced through my head, but most of all, I knew it was not going to be easy to tell her she had a new and potentially significant problem. She was an exacting person who expected treatment with utmost care.

But what she asked me next—no, it was more of a demand—has haunted me all these many years later. It stimulated me to ask questions about our healthcare system that delivers care to people just like her—about the people we work with every day and about how we meet each and every patient's needs to the absolute best of our abilities. I didn't realize at the time that her intriguing request would require new and profound thinking. It would change everything.

"Of course, Dr. Spurlock," she said unapologetically, with certitude, "you'll get me the best cardiologist to deal with this problem."

A reasonable request, impossible to refuse. Why shouldn't she have the best? My response was the expected, "Of course." But I wondered if I was being completely honest.

Who is the "best" cardiologist? How do we really know? Who is the best for heart valve conditions, her likely diagnosis? Doesn't the surgeon matter if or when she needed surgery? She would also need an echocardiogram—was the best-trained and capable person going to read it?

Would she get the best nurses, the best pump technician, the latest technology from the best manufacturers, and the best lab technicians running the many tests she would surely undergo? Would it all happen at the best heart hospital, or at least the best one for new valve conditions? And did it matter that she had other coexisting conditions that the best healthcare clinicians available needed to take into consideration?

Was I truly misleading her if I knew none of the answers to these questions?

But it gets worse. If we could tell through some magical set of transparent, broadly accepted, current performance measures with all of the data for all of the people and systems involved, would I need to find a way to send her to this "best" of all hospitals if it wasn't mine? Doesn't everyone with the same heart valve condition deserve the same best hospital with the best people for his or her condition?

Moreover, what if the "best" place with the best people doesn't have the capacity to handle all of the patients in the country who have a new heart valve issue. Should we prioritize them on a first-come, first-served basis? Do other patients deserve the second best cardiologist or, gasp, "average" care providers?

Could I live with the intellectual dishonesty of knowing that our healthcare system could never help every patient receive care from the "best" cardiologist?

While I'm still struggling with these questions years later, a potential solution is slowly emerging that may answer all of them. It is a radical idea: Everyone has to be the best. Beyond the people, every facility, system, partner and component of healthcare quite simply has to be the best.

Naïve is a word to describe this conclusion. After all, medicine is about probabilities. Traditionally, performance is a bell curve with outliers on both the positive and negative sides. In all of the collaboratives I've ever seen, performance variation is always present, even at the end of the intervention. Nevertheless, striving to make everyone the best seems like the proper, ultimate aim of the collaborative movement—the only solution that makes any sense.

Looking back, the not-so-simple request by a patient with a new heart murmur to see the best cardiologist is the genesis of our mission to make healthcare better, faster and for all patients.

The previous chapters in this book paint a picture of the successful design and execution of collaboratives. Thematically, the authors go beyond simply addressing specific interventions and also describe ways to grow improvement capacity and capability broadly. No collaborative has a goal to create winners and losers among the participants. It is always about everyone being the best—everyone getting better.

In this concluding chapter, we explore the problematic nature of determining the impact of collaboratives and look forward to how the field may evolve over the next several years.

Evaluation Challenge

Understanding the impact of quality improvement programs is challenging, making the rigorous evaluation of large-scale improvement initiatives such as collaboratives herculean.[1,2] A recent systematic review of studies of collaboratives yield mixed or, at best, modest success using evaluation methods that are more traditional.[3] Even less evident are the most crucial aspects of collaboratives.

Now, in this final chapter, following deep insights from some of the best leaders in healthcare with broad experience in designing and running collaboratives, we discover the "science" underpinning the movement is nascent, with some questioning the value of collaboratives.[4]

In this book's foreword, Don Berwick addresses the "messiness" of how and when improvement occurs. The fundamental evaluation challenge in the traditional sense is finding a meaningful "control group" for comparison where an intervention isn't applied. A second challenge is creating specific "variables"—the items being manipulated or evaluated—precisely, ones that don't change over time and are clear enough to apply rigorous statistical analysis. Yet, many authors in this book talk about remaining flexible in the design and operations of the collaborative which creates tension from the rigor required from a traditional evaluation standpoint.

Meaningful Control Groups

Even in the messy world of change and improvement, a traditional quantitative method of evaluation is possible if a control group is available for comparison. A Randomized Controlled Trial (RCT), the bulwark of most diagnostic and treatment studies in healthcare, is ill-suited for improvement initiatives.[5]

Population observational studies, methodologically but still providing some evaluation insight, require comparing "matching controls," and therein lies the rub. The characteristics to "match" are poorly understood.[6] Discussed below in the Collaborative of the Future, the context of improvement often determines the result, and knowing how to control, how to account for, and which contexts matter is at the earliest stages of understanding.

Another line of evaluation coming from the social sciences seeks to understand why something works in some contexts and not others.[7] It abandons the notion of even creating control groups and instead evaluates context, mechanism and outcome in light of a theory of change. It doesn't answer the question, "does it work?" but rather explores both quantitatively and qualitatively why and under what circumstances a program performs well. As we understand context better, this type of evaluation holds promise.

Flexibility vs. Rigor

Another major theme of this book is that a collaborative must continually adapt, within reasonable boundaries, to situations as they occur. Predicting who, when and by how much, and what prompted the change among different participants is folly. Even with deep experience with a change effort, knowing how different participants, especially laggards, respond and the appropriate influence, tools, practices and messages needed to generate action is often trial and error. Yet, it's applied with a basic rigor using rapid cycle testing.

Most traditional research and evaluation, however, requires fixed interventions, with specificity and stability—the antithesis to a flexible "adapt as needed" approach employed by most successful collaboratives. Still, even if a rigorous methodology is possible, using the right combination of variables describing a collaborative, an important question arises around the generalizability of the results. In other words, in our quest to make "everyone the best," not just those in narrowly defined organizations with tightly defined populations, wouldn't broad dissemination still require adapting the lessons from rigorous research? How certain are we that a thoroughly evaluated, evidence-based model is applicable in a variety of different contexts? A major question to answer in the future is, how much fidelity to evidence-based models should exist during implementation in diverse environments?

Persistent Ongoing Evaluation Issues

Many of the contributors to this book identify what some may call "squishy" factors crucial for success. How do you define terms like "community identity," "being part of something bigger than yourself," "peer-to-peer learning," "growing improvement skills," and other social constructs that seemingly evade strict quantitative analysis? Trying to create a "dosing" analysis of meeting attendance or participation in a certain activity to evaluate a collaborative is like checking off a box for "good communication" in an analysis of teamwork. A future challenge is to study many of the important constructs noted in this book using appropriate tools.

Although the problematic nature of evaluation consumes a great deal of time among collaborative leaders, defining what "success" looks like is still plagued with significant challenges. Most use before-and-after comparisons and tools such as statistical process control, which are helpful, but they often paint an incomplete picture. The biggest reason is that collaboratives rarely operate in a vacuum, and several simultaneous exogenous factors may be working to generate change.

For funders who live in the world of finite resources and trade-offs to optimize their impact, these issues are deeply relevant. Collaborative leaders need continually to address the following issues to provide support for the value of collaboratives:

- **Regression to the mean:** Performance tends to improve the most for organizations that are farthest below a population mean and the least for those that are top performers.[8] This is either a result of taking advantage of the "low-hanging fruit," those practices or changes that are easiest to address, or the phenomena of "regression to the mean" or both. Regression to the mean is a function of measurement and not improvement. In other words, what we perceive as change is merely normal variation in a measure's value, and extreme values tend to be less extreme on future measurements. Yet, we often take credit for this type of improvement. And when collaboratives claim victory for moving performance to the mean, the field loses credibility. Moving beyond the "secular" or "background" level of improvement, beyond a larger population mean, is the first mistake to avoid.

- **Opportunity costs:** Could the healthcare system utilize the time, energy and attention spent on collaboratives elsewhere and with greater impact? What are the trade-offs with other programs to accelerate healthcare improvement? How much experimentation and innovation is appropriate with collaboratives or other methods of large-scale change?

  Getting clarity around the opportunity costs is likely a key issue for future growth in the shared learning movement. Moreover, it's possible to find synergistic effects when a variety of approaches and forces are simultaneously applied. Other tools like financial incentives, advocacy/ media pressure, and legal or accreditation mandates may both help and hinder. They likely help when aligned with collaborative issues, but can also compete for attention when worthy topics aren't part of this type of accountability. Future study may be able to tease out when and how the right combination of influences, such as incentives, mandates and voluntary learning is most effective.

- **Sustainability:** What happens after the collaborative is finished? While some collaboratives are ongoing networks or communities for learning, even then, stopping activity on one topic to move to another topic creates the opportunity for backsliding. From an evaluation or even an operational standpoint, there's little research on how to promote quality improvement sustainability. We spend precious resources examining performance three to five years after the conclusion of a large-scale initiative. This is an area in urgent need of thoughtful evaluation.

- **Continual Collaborative Improvement:** Perhaps even more important than whether to utilize a collaborative is the ongoing challenge to continually improve, innovate and expand the impact of shared learning. Using hybrid evaluation methods and idea-sharing platforms like Collaborative Health Network[9] and networking with fellow leaders will promote developing, testing and spreading innovations that help "everyone be the best" faster.

Collaborative of the Future

Have you ever heard someone make a prediction, and by the time the future arrives, the person is long gone or has moved on to new topics? It's amazing how often someone makes a prediction about the future of healthcare and they never evaluate whether the prediction became reality. We definitely need prediction accountability in healthcare. Another way to make a safe prediction is to hedge—to give yourself wiggle room so that almost any eventuality is possible so you can never be wrong—sort of like "the sun will come up tomorrow" type of a prediction. Chaos theory would suggest it's impossible to predict the forces, factors, fads, fashions, drivers, devices, delivery systems, stakeholders, situations, players, providers, plans, purchasers or issues that will dominate the news a year from now, let alone in three to five years. Nevertheless, the following trends have become obvious enough to observe their roles in shared learning programs:

- **Insourcing:** As improvement capacity increases in the system, the need for externally run collaboratives will likely decrease. In other words, organizations of sufficient size and infrastructure are already insourcing collaboratives. If the pace of consolidation and integration in healthcare continues, large organizations will not need external "collaborative experts" to guide their efforts, except perhaps during the early phases of a new innovation. That could leave "external" shared learning to the independent, small, unaffiliated organizations or individuals.

- **Collaborative value:** With increasing use of collaboratives, more people will want to access the same participants. The result is increasing competition among worthy collaboratives. Yet, collaborative fatigue is a real phenomenon. Fatigue comes from complex data burdens, low levels of interaction, inconsistent change packages and improvement too slow to generate excitement. The collaboratives with the most immediate and highest perceived value will squeeze out other worthy programs. As the Connecticut Hospital Association rallies hospitals around their exciting collaborative on High Reliability, as we saw in chapter 7, other topics may not rise to the same level of importance. Competing collaboratives also means that understanding and listening to the participants, the "customers," is invaluable. As a field, prioritizing topics and projects for collaboratives is necessary. But we shouldn't lose the value of local or small-scale regional "laboratories" to test new ideas, emerging topics and innovative learning methods that can grow in scale over time.

The learning and quality improvement projects are all done collaboratively, with clinicians across healthcare settings forming sustainable knowledge and support networks for ongoing improvement.

- **Context:** Understanding local factors, the so-called "context" in which improvement occurs, is a nascent domain in improvement science. It's even

The Champion Model: An Alternative Collaborative

By Karen Wolk Feinstein, Ph.D. and Susan Elster, Ph.D.

In 2005, the Jewish Healthcare Foundation and its Pittsburgh Regional Health Initiative (PRHI) launched the Champions of Work Redesign. The intent was to provide clinical leaders—from multiple and often competing healthcare settings—with the tools and training to improve patient safety and healthcare quality. Traditional collaboratives focus upon deliverables such as specific quality outcomes, cost metrics and survey results that each participant tries to improve. This structure can create winners and losers and can also expose propriety or sensitive information. The champions approach focuses instead on organizational development.

Organized around specific disciplines and competitively selected, successive cohorts have included physicians, nurses, pharmacists, health librarians, paramedics, medical assistants and long-term care providers. A Community Health Worker Champions program is slated to begin in 2016.

Cohorts meet regularly over approximately one year to learn process engineering principles, systems thinking and quality improvement tools via PRHI's Perfecting Patient Care[SM] (PPC) process improvement methodology. They conduct demonstration projects using PPC, receive onsite coaching, and meet with their peers to share experiences and problem-solve together. In a final session, the champions each present the results

challenging to agree on the basic constructs of "context."[10] The saying attributed to statistician George Box that "all models are wrong, but some are useful" touches on the need to explore where adaptation needs to occur.[11] If a major goal of shared learning is to accelerate the spread of useful practices, understanding how, when, where and why to adapt practices, standards, implementation approaches and, yes, healthcare "models" to local situations is crucial to achieve yet more dramatic breakthroughs in care. The question of "fidelity" of a model, or even an evidence-based practice versus local adaptation, is a crucial frontier to explore.

- **Technology:** Technology creates the ability for ad hoc learning. The ease at being able to create multi-channel connections on a moment's notice all over the world speaks to new technology-driven communication vehicles. The democratization of information and shared learning always takes advantage of new ideas and shared learning and is growing right in front of us.

- **New stakeholders:** New partnerships are emerging with patients and families (under the moniker "consumers" when multiple stakeholders are involved) as major players in co-designing and operating collaboratives. Now members of the faith community, retail outlets like Walgreens, salons and barbershops, community networks, not-for-profit local philanthropy groups, and governmental agencies are working together to identify and improve common problems.

Like when predicting the Academy Awards, we project what we think should happen for collaboratives in healthcare (as if we're king or queen for a day and have total control) as well as what's likely to happen, given experience and future trends. Undoubtedly, some of these predictions will not pan out, and in some cases that may be a very good outcome.

High-Priority Improvement Opportunities

What Should Happen: Stratify Interventions by Readiness to Spread

Some topics are complex or tested only in small, homogenous contexts. Other well-developed interventions are successful in diverse settings and have a strong cadre of "early adopters" for peer-to-peer learning. The more complex, uncertain or context-sensitive an intervention or group of interventions is, the more we should first develop "scaling characteristics" to generate more confidence in large-scale spread. Topics or interventions that require a larger portion of an organization for successful implementation, or perhaps multiple organizations, are by their nature more challenging to spread. We need to rapidly explore and understand how, when, why and where to accelerate spread.

of their projects, which are then published to disseminate replicable models for improvement.

Projects include:

Responding to obstetric emergencies (nurse champions)

Eliminating central line infections (physician champions)

Reducing fall risk among elderly psychiatric patients (pharmacist champions)

Developing standardized mass casualty kits – equipment and protocols (EMS champions)

What Will Happen: Popular Issues Get More Attention

Attention by the public or media or policymakers often generates momentum to address dramatic problems, even if less dramatic ones are affecting far more people. Several years ago, addressing Methicillin-Resistant Staphylococcus aureus (MRSA) was hot because of well-covered deaths related to the new "superbug." Over time it became clear that the magnitude of the problem was much less than other important topics yet required a very complex and difficult set of interventions. Later, when hard data out of the Centers for Disease Control and Prevention (CDC) indicated a relatively low disease burden with much less urgency, it fell out of favor as a leading topic to address on a national level.[12] Meanwhile, other topics like severe sepsis and septic shock, with a strong record of accomplishment and huge disease burden due to high mortality rates, flew under the radar. The popular issue dominated the less popular yet more meaningful issue.

Incentives vs. Collaboration

What Should Happen: Promotion of Learning, Mandates/Penalties for Resistant Laggards

There's growing evidence that financial and other incentives have limited impact to accelerate improvement across broad swaths of providers. It's not that they have no role, but "check the box" type mandates or fines for not hitting numbers stimulate gaming, grievance-type advocacy and, worse, limited improvement on outcomes.[13] In an environment of shared learning like in our collaboratives, soft competition (where personal pride drives performance) and critical mass "can't be left behind" social motivation, large groups of healthcare providers can and have dramatically accelerated improvement with many examples in this book alone. Unfortunately, the reality is that not everyone is on board even with collaboratives; some need gentle nudging and others only respond to hammers such that the group of laggard participants is likely where penalties have the biggest impact. Shared learning first, penalties for the recalcitrant.

What Will Happen: Accountability First, Social Motivation Later

When I attended a meeting of nearly 1,000 diverse healthcare stakeholders, a representative from a Fortune 500 company went to the microphone and proclaimed that authorities would have indicted and jailed his CEO if he allowed as many errors as hospital CEOs allowed hospital-acquired infections. And while he doesn't speak for all, the notion of addressing systems as the main leverage point for improvement instead of disciplining people with predictable human frailties ("to err is human") has not made it out of the "inside baseball" crowd of healthcare. Calls for accountability in the face of seemingly preventable errors still dominate the debate. Some commentators and industry leaders also view financial rewards and penalties as the dominant drivers of change in spite of the underwhelming experience to date and extensive research in motivational theory. But the voices are loud and create a powerful narrative that drowns out the more difficult to understand power of social and professional motivation that works so well with collaboratives.

New Opportunities with Heightened Competition

What Should Happen: Collaboration on Social Determinants of Care

Collaboratives always have a foundation of working together for common goals as a necessary starting point for shared learning. This usually translates into generally non-competitive topics. When was the last time you saw a healthcare billboard promoting an organization as the one with the fewest complications? Yet, as consolidation and integration increase in response to a transforming healthcare system, coupled with a growing emphasis on payment incentives based on relative performance, growing competitiveness will exclude ever more topics that previously were ripe targets for collaborative learning. A topic that should grow in importance is collective and collaborative action addressing the social determinants of care, even among competing organizations.

What Will Happen: Collaboration on Social Determinants of Care

If healthcare really expands from a one-case-at-a-time service industry to include caring for populations that are both well (with or without chronic conditions) and sick, addressing all of the factors that limit wellness will receive new and growing attention. Even in highly competitive environments, and with a nod to herd immunity, cooperation on social determinants of care seems almost too obvious. If neighbors in poor communities are connected to different organizations, working collaboratively to provide systems and practices to the entire community independent of which organization is accountable is likely to benefit all.

Future Collaborative Approaches

What Should Happen: Prioritization of Variables for Study and Testing Based on Consensus

A challenging aspect for better understanding the context where different initiatives flourish and where they fail is the lack of a clear taxonomy or a set of consensus terms useful for evaluation. From the methodologist standpoint, what factors to operationalize, measure and control are foundational, yet little agreement exists on these factors.[14] A good example is leadership engagement, an important variable with face validity. Yet, efforts to quantify leadership engagement objectively have not yet attained consensus. If we systematically evaluate high-priority contextual topics, the field will more quickly understand how to apply them and reach desired outcomes.

What Will Happen: Both Local Improvisation and Formal Research

Social-science-based research methodologies will likely dominate our understanding of how to spread useful ideas. It's probable that new ways to test innovation will also grow and we will gain insights on how to take local context better into consideration.[15] Adapting for local context is akin to modifying an original piece of music. A musical arrangement adapts the musical content for different instruments, voices or settings but keeps the essence and main features of the score. Musical improvisation adds new creativity and innovation but requires substantial talent to be effective. Formal and informal learning are useful constructs that will guide future collaboratives.

New Methods of Shared Learning

What Should Happen: New Forms of Shared Learning

Collaboration—there's an app for that! People will invariably innovate on ways to convene, share ideas and learn faster with new technologies. Groups are already organizing across organizations, countries, even continents, to explore and test ideas.

What Will Happen: Exciting New Forms of Shared Learning

Shared learning will never vanish—it's how people are built. Healthcare teams and organizations will find a way to address common issues, with new partnerships and expanding tools to communicate. The translation of research evidence, data from measurement, and adapting practices in different settings will drive new forms of learning, with committed, collaboratively oriented leaders. In fact, one purpose of this book is to catalyze new forms of shared learning and to spread many other creative ways humans learn from and with each other.

Conclusion

If you're reading this book and designing or running a healthcare collaborative, or perhaps considering it, you carry an enormous responsibility to help everyone be the best. If you're working in a healthcare field that in some way ultimately gets care to patients and families, you carry an enormous responsibility to make sure each of them receives the best possible care. If you're training, building, inventing, regulating, funding, accrediting, marketing or researching, or are in any way connected with healthcare you share the same responsibility: Humanity dictates that each person deserves the best.

Words like "daunting," "provocative," "exciting," "worthy" and "meaningful" all describe the challenge collaboratives face. They must remain dynamic, focusing on the big picture aims and also with attention to the tiniest of operational details. In a continual state of learning, collaboratives must inspire, adapt and retain steel-like resolve about the importance of their task.

We hope that you've found in this book answers to your questions, or ideas to test, or a new insight that stimulates a change in course. With our first collaborative in the late '90s on patient experience, to the thriving Beacon—Bay Area Patient Safety Collaborative with 38 committed hospitals and an involved funder like the Gordon & Betty Moore Foundation—to the ongoing national Partnership for Patients program, we're learning that a little discomfort and uncertainty is the price of admission. The work is never truly done. We have too much to improve in healthcare to say we're finished improving, but the rewards are plentiful. Participating in improvement is a terrific anti-burnout treatment. It creates its own sense of meaning and greater joy when sharing it with friends and colleagues.

Designing or running a collaborative takes you out of your comfort zone. This is where we explore, where we innovate, where we fail, and often through tenacity and persistence, we also succeed. It's where the good life begins. You likely detected the palpable excitement, the joy, the desire to share and the fabulous stories that more than 40 international contributors made in the pages of this book. The question is, then, are you "All In?"

---

[1] Berwick, DM. "The Science of Improvement." *JAMA* 299, no. 10 (March 2008): 1182-4.

[2] Berwick, DM. "The Question of Improvement." *JAMA* 307, no. 19 (2012): 20093-94.

[3] de Silva, D. *No. 21 Improvement collaboratives in health care.* Report, London: The Health Foundation, 2014.

[4] Pronovost P, Jha AK. "Did Hospital Engagement Networks Actually Improve Care?" *NEJM* 371, no. 4 (August 2014): 691-3.

[5] Davidoff, F. "Improvement Interventions are Social Treatments, Not Pills." *Ann Intern Med.* 161, no. 7 (October 2014): 526-7.

[6] Shekelle PG, et al. "Advancing the Science of Patient Safety." *Ann Intern Med.* 154, no. 10 (May 2011): 693-6.

[7] Marchal, B, S Van Belle, G Westhorp, and G Peersman. *Realist Evaluation.* http://betterevaluation.org/approach/realist_evaluation (accessed September 5, 2015).

[8] Spurlock, B, R Abravanel, and S Spurlock. *Do Hospital Characterisitcs Drive Clinical Performance?* Report, Oakland: California HealthCare Foundation, 2008.

[9] *Collaborative Health Network.* healthdoers.bravenew.com.

[10] Agency for Healthcare Research and Quality. "Making Health Care Safer II." *www.ahrq.gov.* March 1, 2013. http://www.ahrq.gov/sites/default/files/wysiwyg/research/findings/evidence-based-reports/services/quality/ptsafetysum.pdf (accessed September 5, 2015).

[11] Box, GE, and NR Draper. *Empirical Model-Building and Response Surfaces.* Wiley, 1987.

[12] Dudeck, MA, LM Weiner, PJ Malpiedi, and et al. "Risk Adjustment ofr Healthcare Facility-Onset C. difficile and MRSA Bacteremia in NHSN." *Center for Disease Control and Prevention.* March 12, 2013. http://www.cdc.gov/nhsn/pdfs/mrsa-cdi/RiskAdjustment-MRSA-CDI.pdf (accessed September 9, 2015).

[13] Damberg, C, et al. "Measuring Success in Health Care Value-Based Purchasing Programs." *www.rand.org.* 2014. www.rand.org/pubs/research_reports/RR306 (accessed September 5, 2015).

[14] Agency for Healthcare Research and Quality. "Making Health Care Safer II." *www.ahrq.gov.* March 1, 2013. http://www.ahrq.gov/sites/default/files/wysiwyg/research/findings/evidence-based-reports/services/quality/ptsafetysum.pdf (accessed September 5, 2015).

[15] Asch, DA, and R Rosin. "Innovation as Discipline, Not Fad." *NEJM* 373, no. 7 (August 2015): 592-4.

ABOUT THE AUTHORS

Ken Alexander, MS, RRT, VP, Louisiana Hospital Association (Chapter 7)
Mr. Alexander is responsible for leading Louisiana Hospital Association's quality and patient safety initiatives, assisting member hospitals statewide with issues relative to regulatory and hospital licensing standards and activities.

Gail Amundson, M.D., Healthcare Transformation Consultant (Chapter 11)
Dr. Amundson is an advisor to The Alliance on QualityPath™ initiative for high-value orthopedic and cardiac care; and consultant to business, government and healthcare clients on healthcare policy, quality improvement and healthcare system redesign.

Pierre M. Barker, MD., Institute for Healthcare Improvement (IHI) (Chapter 2)
Dr. Barker is the Senior Vice President responsible IHI's large-scale health systems improvement initiatives outside the USA.

James B. Battles, Ph.D., Social Science Analyst, AHRQ/CQuiPS (Chapter 9)
Dr. Battles leads AHRQ's efforts in the assessment of patient safety culture, and improving teamwork (TeamSTEPPS®) in collaboration with the Department of Defense.

Donald M. Berwick, M.D., President Emeritus and Senior Fellow, Institute for Healthcare Improvement (Chapter 2)

Dr. Berwick has published more than 110 scientific articles in numerous professional journals on subjects relating to healthcare policy, decision analysis, technology assessment, and healthcare quality management.

Bruce Block, M.D., Chief Medical Informatics Officer and Chief Learning Officer, Jewish Healthcare Foundation (Chapter 10)

Dr. Block supports healthcare innovations designed to effectively use evidence, improve processes and influence behavior.

Jane Brock, M.D., MSPH, Medical Director, Telligen (Chapter 6)

Dr. Brock currently serves as the clinical director of the Quality Innovation Network (QIN)-Quality Improvement Organization (QIO) National Coordinating Center (NCC), funded by CMS.

Daniel Buffington, Pharm.D., MBA, Clinical Pharmacology Services, Inc. (Chapter 4)

Dr. Buffington has served as a leader in interdisciplinary efforts to improve practice models, clinical documentation, and electronic health records systems to ensure the accuracy and effectiveness of collaborative medication management.

Jason Byrd, J.D., Director of Patient Safety and Director of the Hospital Engagement Network (HEN), Carolinas HealthCare System (Chapters 1, 11)

Mr. Byrd's prior work includes developing and leading the D2B (Door-to-Balloon): An Alliance for Quality campaign, which focused on reducing D2B times for STEMI patients through implementation of evidence-based strategies in 1,100 hospitals worldwide.

Jim Chase, President, MNCommunity Measurement (Chapter 11)

Mr. Chase has more than 25 years of experience in healthcare management; he's a nationally recognized expert on performance measurement and healthcare transparency.

John B. Chessare M.D., MPH (Chapter 10)

Dr. Chessare has been actively involved in designing and managing systems of care in academic medical centers and in community hospitals.

Jim Conway, MS, LFACHE, Adjunct Faculty, Harvard T.H. Chan School of Public Health (Chapter 12)

Mr. Conway's areas of expertise and interest include governance and executive leadership, patient safety, change management, crisis management and patient-/family-centered care.

Andrew Cooper, Interim Director of Communications, Public Health Wales (Chapter 13)

Mr. Cooper has over twenty years communications experience, working across the public, private and third sectors. He served as the head of communications for the 1000 Lives Improvement service in NHS Wales, developing the role of communications in the field of quality improvement.

Mary Cooper, M.D., J.D., Chief Quality Officer and VP, Quality and Safety, Connecticut Hospital Association (Chapter 7)

Dr. Cooper oversees the implementation of High Reliability Science Connecticut hospitals, CHA's Partnership for Patients (with AHA/HRET), hospital value creation with their quality and safety strategy, and working closely with the state government and quality organizations.

Susan Elster, Ph.D., Research Director, JHF and PRHI (Chapter 14)

Dr. Elster is a consultant to the Jewish Healthcare Foundation and its supporting organizations; she has expertise in project development and research design, with an emphasis on survey and focus group methodology and strategic planning.

Jo Ann Endo, MSW, Content Development Manager, Institute for Healthcare Improvement (Chapter 13)

Ms. Endo specializes in creating original content for the IHI website, including writing blog posts and conducting video interviews.

Karen Wolk Feinstein, Ph.D., President and CEO, Jewish Healthcare Foundation and Pittsburgh Regional Health Initiative (Chapters 10, 12, 14)

Dr. Feinstein is regarded as a national leader in healthcare quality improvement and frequently presents at national and international conferences.

Brianna Gass, MPH, Lead Program Evaluator, Telligen (Chapter 6)

Ms. Gass is experienced in program evaluation, facilitates evaluation activities of Quality Improvement Organizations (QIOs), and conducts evaluation of other national and community-based healthcare quality improvement efforts.

Stephen Hines, Ph.D., Chief Research Officer, Health Research and Educational Trust (Chapter 9)

Dr. Hines helps to lead and plan large-scale improvement initiatives and oversees HRET analytic work that examines why some participants in these projects make great progress while others do not.

Alison L. Hong, M.D., Director, Quality and Patient Safety, Connecticut Hospital Association (Chapter 7)

Dr. Hong has been the project lead on numerous collaboratives at the state and national level including On the CUSP: Stop BSI and the Partnership for Patients.

Libby Hoy, Founder/CEO, PFCCpartners (Chapter 12)

Libby Hoy has 20+ years of raising three boys with Mitochondrial disease as well as years of experience in bringing together all healthcare stakeholders in partnership to create sustainable improvement in healthcare.

Andrea Kabcenell, RN, MPH, VP, Institute for Healthcare Improvement (Chapter 9)

Ms. Kabcenell serves as a lead on the IHI's Innovation Team, driving and developing projects from innovative ideas to practice implementation; her role also assures that new knowledge is used in IHI and other programs.

Jenny Kowalczuk, writer/researcher, www.jennykowalczuk.co.uk, Hyderus (Chapter 13)

Ms. Kowalczuk is a writer and researcher specializing in public and global health; she has an MA in human science and works independently with NGOs, government and commercial clients.

Elizabeth (Betsy) A. Lee, MSPH, BSN, RN, President, BL Enterprises, LLC, Patient Safety/Quality Improvement Consultant (Chapter 7)

Ms. Lee is a consultant to New Hope of Indiana and to Indiana University School of Nursing for interprofessional collaborative practice; her prior role included providing leadership, education and strategic direction for the Indiana Patient Safety Center (IPSC).

Deneil LoGiudice, Consultant, Continuous Improvement (Chapter 11)
Ms. LoGiudice is a quality improvement consultant currently working with multiple nonprofit organizations; she has a background in quality engineering and holds a Lean Six Sigma Black Belt certification from American Society for Quality (ASQ).

Virginia A. McBride, RN, MPH, Organ Transplantation Regulatory and Performance Improvement Consultant (Chapter 13)
Ms. McBride provides transplantation performance improvement, regulatory compliance, and interim staffing services, such as interim transplant administrator to transplant hospitals.

Joe McCannon, Co-founder and Principal, The Billions Institute (Chapter 1)
Mr. McCannon leads international nonprofits that serve movements, foundations and organizations—across social sectors—to expand impact to massive scale.

Paul McGann, M.D., Chief Medical Officer for Quality Improvement, Co-Director, Partnership for Patients Co-Director, Transforming Clinical Practices Initiative, Centers for Medicare & Medicaid Services (Chapter 4)
Dr. McGann's first projects at CMS were to lead the introduction of quality improvement work in nursing homes and home health agencies into the Quality Improvement Organization contracts (published in the Annals of Internal Medicine in September 2006).

Kevin O'Connor, President and CEO, LifeCenter Northwest (Chapter 7)
Mr. O'Connor has served as President and CEO of LifeCenter Northwest (LCNW), the OPO serving Washington, Montana, Alaska and Northern Idaho. Under his leadership organ donation at LCNW has increased by 65 percent, and tissue donation has more than quadrupled.

Christopher Queram, MA, President/CEO, Wisconsin Collaborative for Healthcare Quality (WCHQ) (Chapter 7)
Mr. Queram has been the president and CEO of the Wisconsin Collaborative for Healthcare Quality—a voluntary consortium of organizations working to improve the quality and affordability of healthcare in Wisconsin.

Lucy A. Savitz, Ph.D., MBA, Assistant VP, Delivery System Science, Institute for Healthcare Leadership, Intermountain Healthcare; Research Professor, Epidemiology, University of Utah; Discovery & Dissemination Board Committee Chair, High Value Healthcare Collaborative (Chapter 5)

Dr. Savitz leads the Intermountain-based ACTION III network, directs the CMMI Innovation Challenge award, and serves on the Board representing Discovery and Dissemination for the High Value Health Care Collaborative.

John Scanlon, Ph.D., Partner, Financial Transformations, Inc. (Chapter 4)
Dr. Scanlon designs leadership campaigns that enable executive teams to take their organizations through strategic transformation.

Marybeth Sharpe, Ph.D., Program Director, Gordon and Betty Moore Foundation (Chapter 9)
Dr. Sharpe directs the Gordon and Betty Moore Foundation's regional healthcare improvement initiatives, including a 10+ years effort to improve hospital patient safety and care transitions in Northern California; in this role, she collaborates with local partners and national stakeholders to advance the role of frontline RNs in measurably improving patient care outcomes.

Michael P. Silver, MPH, SVP, Improvement Science and Consulting Services, HealthInsight (Chapter 6)
Mr. Silver has been engaged in the design, conduct, and analysis of healthcare quality improvement and patient safety initiatives for more than 20 years; he provides technical assistance to healthcare innovations projects in all settings, with a broad range of targets, across the country.

Bruce W. Spurlock, M.D., Executive Director, Cynosure Health (Chapter 14)
Dr. Spurlock is the co-editor for this book as well as the executive director of Cynosure Health; his primary responsibility is to direct and facilitate large, multi-participant healthcare quality collaboratives designed to accelerate the dissemination of evidence-based clinical practices.

Diane Stewart, MBA, Senior Director, Pacific Business Group on Health (Chapter 5)
Ms. Stewart was a founding member, and now Board member, for the Network for Regional Health Improvement, a national organization of multi-stakeholder regional health initiatives to promote transparency and system improvement across local healthcare systems.

Sarah M. Stout, MPAff, Managing Consultant, The Lewin Group (Chapter 8)
Ms. Stout brings more than 10 years' experience in project management, collaborative design and implementation, strategic planning, stakeholder engagement, and qualitative and quantitative research.

Patricia A. Teske, RN, MHA, Implementation Officer, Cynosure Health (Introduction, Chapter 3)
Ms. Teske is the co-editor for this book and is working to implement Cynosure's vision through strategic planning and execution of projects on time and within budget that yield success.

Jeff Thompson, M.D., Executive Advisor and Chief Executive Officer Emeritus, Gunderson Health System (Chapter 3)
Dr. Thompson has served on Gundersen's boards beginning in 1992 and played a key role in the organization's negotiations and governance design.

Dennis Wagner, MPA, Director, Quality Improvement and Innovation Group, Centers for Medicare and Medicaid Services (Chapter 4)
Mr. Wagner is a national and international leader in the fields of healthcare quality improvement, the environment and social marketing; he's a thoughtful and strategic person who believes in committing to and delivering on bold aims in work and life.

Sam R. Watson, MSA, CPPS, Senior VP Patient Safety and Quality, Michigan Health & Hospital Association (Chapter 5)
Mr. Watson oversaw the national launch of the core measures clinical data collection system; led the inauguration of statewide quality initiatives, and achieved the Eisenberg Innovation in Patient Safety and Quality Award and the Dick Davidson Quality Milestone Award for healthcare improvement.

Alan Willson, Ph.D., Improvement Consultant, Aneurin Bevan Health Board, South Wales (Chapter 13)
Dr. Willson is a senior research officer in the Improvement Science Research Group at the College of Human and Health Sciences, Swansea University.

Nancy D. Zionts, MBA, Chief Operating Officer/Chief Program Officer, Jewish Healthcare Foundation (Chapter 12)
Ms. Zionts is responsible for the grant agenda for the Foundation and its operating arms, the Pittsburgh Regional Health Initiative and Health Careers Futures as the COO/Chief Program Officer for the Jewish Healthcare Foundation.

ACKNOWLEDGEMENTS

As we state in the Introduction, the "thing speaks for itself." This book is the culmination of tens or maybe even hundreds of thousands of hours of experience by the 40 contributors, their colleagues, and partners who have designed and run collaboratives.

As we assembled this book, we wanted to replicate the collaborative spirit that we witness every day. Each writer's ideas are crucial to a comprehensive review of the subject, and there were also many more contributors behind the scenes that we'd like to thank and acknowledge.

At the outset, we wish to thank Marybeth Sharpe, with whom we've worked for the past decade on a variety of patient safety grants; Heather Rosett, our program officer for this book; and Delphine Henri, who guided us in communication and dissemination strategies. They helped us conceive, fund, cheerlead, problem solve and guide the project throughout our journey.

Additionally, we thank the entire team from the Gordon and Betty Moore Foundation and the staff, past and present, who supported and taught us along the way: Helen Kim, George Bo-Linn, Karyn DiGiorgio, Liz Malcolm, Amy Mushlin, Martha Nicholson, Diane Schweitzer, Brenda Stone, Katie Ward and Kate Weiland. The Foundation has always been a visionary, intellectual partner and funder from the first BEACON—The Bay Area Patient Safety Collaborative in 2005 to the present. This book is strong evidence of the tremendous impact the Foundation has in the San Francisco Bay Area, which is now spreading across the country and even internationally.

Special thanks go to our colleagues at Cynosure Health: Marsha Chan, Missy Peters, Linda Langel and Samantha Spurlock. They organized and coordinated thousands of logistical activities, meetings, contributor connections, advisory group members, end notes and many other details. They were the "glue" to a very complex project and we're permanently indebted for their work, encouragement and sound advice. We'd also like to thank the entire Cynosure Health team with whom we've had the pleasure of designing and running several collaboratives, including Kathleen Carrothers, Gerald Clute, Jackie Conrad, Barb DeBaun, Lisa Ehle, Kathy Fleming, Christine Muscolo, Michael Purvis, Cheryl Ruble, Jennifer Stockey, Steve Tremain, Kim Werkmeister and Maryanne Whitney. Our work together greatly influences this book.

Despite our experience designing and running collaboratives, our knowledge of editing a multi-chapter book was lacking. We reached out to experts and are very grateful for their guidance. We want to thank Lee Gutkind for his sage advice and tough feedback, and Michael Zirulnik for his support, kindness and exemplary fact checking. We would also like to thank Arian Dasmalchi for her editing and patience with our occasional version-control issues. We're grateful for the logistical, graphic design and style advice we received from Sarah Starke and Anthony Puttee as well.

One of the best parts of the project was an advisory group of senior leaders in healthcare improvement who are deeply engaged in healthcare transformation. They took time out to convene and direct the overall book strategy. The advisory group represents diverse perspectives, recommended all of our contributors, and helped us address core principles and simultaneously innovate. They include Anne-Marie Audet at United Hospital Fund, James Battles at Agency for Healthcare Research & Quality (AHRQ), Marc Bennett at HealthInsight, Mary Dixon-Woods at University of Leicester, Tom Evans at Iowa Healthcare Collaborative, Helen Haskell at Mothers Against Medical Error, Steve Hines at Health Research & Educational Trust, Hillary Jalon at United Hospital Fund, Andrea Kabcenell at Institute for Healthcare Improvement,

Paul McGann at CMS/CCSQ, Harold Miller at Center for Healthcare Quality and Payment Reform, Gary Oftedahl formerly with the Institute for Clinical Systems Improvement, Peter Pronovost at John Hopkins Medicine, Michael McGinnis at Institute of Medicine, Chris Queram at Wisconsin Collaborative for Health Care Quality, Roger Resar at Institute for Healthcare Improvement, Heather Rosett at Betty Irene Moore Nursing Initiative, Marybeth Sharpe at Betty Irene Moore Nursing Initiative and Betty Irene Moore School of Nursing, Diane Stewart at Pacific Business Group on Health, Dennis Wagner at CMS/CCSQ, Sam Watson at Michigan Keystone, and Karen Wolk Feinstein at Jewish Healthcare Foundation.

Particular thanks go to Brent James at Intermountain Healthcare for his guidance on several critical issues and constructing the back cover note, and to Joe McCannon at Billions Institute who received multiple timely calls about optimizing the topics and asking for assistance managing specific issues.

Several of our advisors served as contributors and/or offered recommendations about individuals they believed would add a valuable voice to this effort. Each contributor also relied on colleagues to read, edit, suggest and support their individual work. It's amazing how quickly the list expands with all the people who helped during the project. Although we likely don't know all of them, a few we want to acknowledge are Molly Lunn, Jane Roessner, John Scanlon, Dan Schummers and Valerie Weber.

We were also guided in this effort by the voice of the customer, and gratefully acknowledge the time and suggestions provided during interviews with the following individuals: Jessica Blake, Jeanne Conry, Angela Herrick, Tom Jackson, Helen Macfie, Barbara Murphy, Diane Radigan, Michael Silver and Ana Torres.

Another lesson that becomes obvious when you run a collaborative is that you usually learn the most from the participants themselves. We've gained more insights, practical experience and valuable lessons from our first program on patient experience with California Hospitals, through the

BEACON collaborative, Washington State Safe Tables, Southern California Patient Safety Collaborative, Florida Readmissions and Surgical Care Initiatives, Patient Safety First initiative, Avoid Readmissions through Collaboration (ARC) Collaborative, Safety Net Institute DSRIP collaborative, Clinical Improvement Interest Groups and the nearly 1,500 hospitals, 31 State Hospital Associations with the Hospital Engagement Network led by Maulik Joshi, Charisse Coloumbe and team at the Healthcare Research and Education Trust (HRET).

Finally, neither of us could have finished the project without the strong encouragement, patience, words of wisdom and often humor as a way to keep everything in proper perspective from our spouses: Chris Teske and Shelley Spurlock.

A collaborative always starts with a common goal along with shared experience and learning from many participants. *All In: Using Healthcare Collaboratives to Save Lives and Improve Care* emulates that truism, and we're deeply thankful for so many participants.

CPSIA information can be obtained
at www.ICGtesting.com
Printed in the USA
LVOW10s2058100717
540826LV00032B/1221/P

9 780996 792707